PSYCHIATRIC RESEARCH IN AMERICA

This is a volume in the Arno Press collection

HISTORICAL ISSUES IN MENTAL HEALTH

Advisory Editor
Gerald N. Grob

Editorial Board
David Mechanic
Jacques M. Quen
Charles E. Rosenberg

See last pages of this volume for a complete list of titles

PSYCHIATRIC RESEARCH IN AMERICA

Two Studies 1936-1941

Edited by
Gerald N. Grob

ARNO PRESS

A New York Times Company
New York • 1980

St. Philip's College Library

616.89
N277 ps
1980

Editorial Supervision: Brian Quinn

Reprint Edition 1980 by Arno Press Inc.
HISTORICAL ISSUES IN MENTAL HEALTH
ISBN for complete set: 0-405-11900-3
See last pages of this volume for titles.
Manufactured in the United States of America

Library of Congress Cataloging in Publication Data

National Committee for Mental Hygiene.
    Psychiatric research in America.

    (Historical issues in mental health)
    Reprint of the 1938 ed. of Research in mental hospi-
tals ... 1936-1937, and of the 1942 ed. of Research in
mental hospitals, study number two ... 1939-1941, both
published by the Committee, New York.
    1. Psychiatric research--United States. 2. Psychi-
atric hospitals--United States. I. Grob, Gerald N.,
1931-   II. National Committee for Mental Hygiene.
Research in mental hospitals. III. Title. IV. Series.
RC337.N32 1979   616.8'9'0072073   78-22583
ISBN 0-405-11931-3

St. Philip's College Library

CONTENTS

69631

RESEARCH IN MENTAL HOSPITALS

A Survey and Tentative Appraisal of Research Activities,
Facilities and Possibilities in State Hospitals
and Other Tax-Supported Institutions for
the Mentally Ill and Defective in the
United States

Conducted by

The National Committee for Mental Hygiene

1936-1937

Field Representatives
CHARLES P. FITZPATRICK, M.D., *Clinical Director,*
Butler Hospital, Providence, R. I.

WINFRED OVERHOLSER, M.D., *Supt.,*
St. Elizabeths Hospital, Washington, D. C.;
formerly Massachusetts Commissioner for Mental Disease

Assisted by
SAMUEL W. HAMILTON, M.D., *Director,*
Mental Hospital Survey Committee
JOSEPH ZUBIN, PH.D., *Statistician,*
Mental Hospital Survey Committee
PAUL O. KOMORA, *Associate Secretary,*
The National Committee for Mental Hygiene

Advisory Committee

Clarence O. Cheney, M.D., Chairman
Kenneth E. Appel, M.D.
Karl M. Bowman, M.D.
Adolf Meyer, M.D.

Joseph E. Raycroft, M.D.
H. Douglas Singer, M.D.
William J. Tiffany, M.D.
C. Fred Williams, M.D.

Ex-Officio Members
Samuel W. Hamilton, M.D.
Clarence M. Hincks, M.D.
Nolan D. C. Lewis, M.D.
Arthur H. Ruggles, M.D.

THE NATIONAL COMMITTEE FOR MENTAL HYGIENE, INC.
50 WEST 50TH ST.,
NEW YORK CITY

St. Philip's College Library

COPYRIGHT, 1938, BY
THE NATIONAL COMMITTEE FOR MENTAL HYGIENE, INC.

Printed in the United States of America by
BOYD PRINTING COMPANY, ALBANY, N. Y.

FOREWORD

There is a growing conviction in America that the problems presented by mental disorders will become more and more acute unless adequate arrangements are made for the prosecution of research to point the way to more effective programs of prevention and treatment. While mental hospitals and clinics are essential, there is little prospect of materially reducing the burden of mental illness by the mere multiplication of such facilities. At the present time, according to the American Medical Association, the mental institutions of the United States are providing care for 546,906 patients on a daily average and thousands of additional patients are provided for through out-patient clinics. The demands for these services are increasing each year. To meet current needs a 20 per cent increase in mental hospital accommodation and a doubling of out-patient clinics are required. When these deficiencies have been met there will be the expectation next year, and the years to follow, of additional demands for increased services. Such a prospect is not encouraging. Mental hospitalization costs now exceed $200,000,000 a year and large increments may prove embarrassing to the taxpayer.

The possibility, through research, of altering the existing trend of mounting hospital and clinic loads is indeed great. In this connection we are reminded of the brilliant results that have been achieved in connection with general paresis—a condition that once accounted for 10 per cent of admissions to mental hospitals and that proved invariably fatal. Today, because of scientific research, the ravages of this disease have become materially reduced. And there are grounds for optimism in dealing more effectively with dementia praecox which is responsible for the occupancy of 50 per cent of mental hospital beds. Experimental work with insulin shock and metrazol has opened avenues for the scientific study of this disease that will probably lead to a larger measure of control. The introduction of the electro-encephalograph could be cited as furnishing a further basis for the hope of making signal advances through research in connection with psychiatric problems.

With the aim of contributing to progress in the mental hygiene field the present study was undertaken. It presents for the first time an outline picture of the research situation in tax-supported institutions for the mentally ill and defective, and gives us a clearer appreciation of the extent and quality of existing scientific endeavor, of the number of qualified men engaged in investigative work, of the problems that hamper the extension of psychiatric research, and of the promising leads to future scientific progress in these institutions. It provides a factual basis which will serve as a point of departure and orientation and, we trust, as a stimulus toward the further and more rapid development of research interest and activity in public mental hospitals. As such we hope it will prove of interest and value to hospital executives, hospital trustees, legislatures, budget-making bodies and other governmental authorities, and to Foundations and Funds who are turning their attention and financial support increasingly to this promising field of medical science.

The report is divided into five parts. Part I gives "the gist of it," in which the major findings and conclusions of the study may be seen at a glance. Part II interprets the findings as they concern state hospitals especially, since these institutions form the backbone of public provisions for the care and treatment of the mentally ill in the United States and are the center of interest of our study in the main. Part III describes the research activities and facilities in the principal hospital centers. It is perhaps the most significant section of the report, disclosing, as it does, the impressive character and extent of scientific work already under way or projected in tax-supported mental hospitals. They are the pivotal centers to which we must look for encouragement, guidance and leadership in extending psychiatric research to other institutions. Part IV presents a statistical analysis of our findings, in which an attempt has been made to measure, as objectively as possible, the clinical factors that enter basically into a determination of a hospital's fitness for research work. It is of fundamental importance to the whole study, for sound and effective scientific work depends crucially on superior standards of clinical work, and the appraisal of potential capacity for research activity involves necessarily an evaluation of clinical standards. Part V contains rating scales, geographical data, and other supplementary information pertinent to the study.

The John and Mary R. Markle Foundation furnished the financial support for this undertaking and has generously funded a further survey in connection with privately supported hospitals and institutions. The reports of both studies will give a comprehensive picture of the present status of psychiatric research in the United States.

The National Committee for Mental Hygiene is indebted not only to the John and Mary R. Markle Foundation but also to a distinguished group of psychiatrists and administrators who gave material assistance in planning and conducting this survey.

CLARENCE M. HINCKS, M.D.

General Director,
The National Committee for Mental Hygiene

TABLE OF CONTENTS

PART V

PART I

SUMMARY AND CONCLUSIONS

Part I

Summary and Conclusions

Origin of Survey

IN April, 1936, the John and Mary R. Markle Foundation made a grant to The National Committee for Mental Hygiene for the purpose of studying the research possibilities of state hospitals and other tax-supported institutions for the care and treatment of the mentally ill. The study was to be in the nature of an "orientation" survey—a canvass of existing research arrangements and trends in publicly supported hospital systems; a focusing of attention on centers that are worthy of emulation by other hospitals; the discovery, if possible, of hospitals that offer significant opportunities for the further development of research programs; the discovery of staff members of public institutions who have been demonstrating a genuine interest in research, with a capacity for investigatory effort; the determination of the degree of liaison that exists between mental hospitals and medical schools or other scientific centers; and, finally, the consideration of practical steps that might be taken to encourage and promote sound research developments in this field.

Significance of Research in Public Institutions

The appropriateness of looking to our publicly supported hospitals for investigatory work is evident when we take into account the vast patient populations now resident in these hospitals that offer unrivalled opportunities for observation and study. And in contributing to an enlargement of knowledge in the psychiatric field, staff members become imbued with a scientific spirit that is reflected in better clinical work. It is a matter of observation that without research, any clinical group of workers

3

tends to drift into a scholastic attitude in which the opinions of former authorities are substituted for actual observation and frequent reorientation. On the other hand medical groups that have one or more members working on some research project are stimulated to a greater alertness and usefulness to their patients. It is also worthy of note that the task of recruiting promising men for mental hospital posts is facilitated if there can be held out the inducements of clinical work that is not routinized and, in addition, opportunities for investigatory efforts.

SCOPE AND METHOD OF SURVEY

In determining the scope of the survey, it was decided to give a wide interpretation to the term "tax-supported" —including under this designation all hospitals for the mentally ill supported entirely by public funds—federal, state, county and city—as well as public institutions for the care of epileptics and the feebleminded. Privately owned or endowed hospitals were not included in the list even though they accepted patients maintained by public funds.

Plans for the survey were formulated with the assistance of an advisory committee composed of* representative leaders in the mental hospital field, and methods of study were devised with due regard for economy in time and expense, considering the requirements of the broad canvass projected. Field work was begun under the active direction of Dr. Charles P. Fitzpatrick of Butler Hospital, Providence, R. I., and carried through the summer and fall of 1936, with the timely assistance of a selected group of

* Dr. Kenneth E. Appel, Institute of the Pennsylvania Hospital; Dr. Karl M. Bowman, Director, Psychiatric Division, Bellevue Hospital; Dr. Clarence O. Cheney, Director, Westchester Division, New York Hospital; Dr. Adolf Meyer, Director, Henry Phipps Psychiatric Clinic; Dr. Joseph E. Raycroft, New Jersey Department of Institutions and Agencies; Dr. H. Douglas Singer, Director, Illinois Psychiatric Institute; Dr. William J. Tiffany, New York State Commissioner of Mental Hygiene; and Dr. C. Fred Williams, Superintendent, South Carolina State Hospital. Ex-officio members, Dr. Samuel W. Hamilton, Director, Mental Hospital Survey Committee; Dr. Clarence M. Hincks, General Director, The National Committee for Mental Hygiene; Dr. Nolan D. C. Lewis, Director, New York State Psychiatric Institute; and Dr. Arthur H. Ruggles, Director, Butler Hospital.

hospital psychiatrists whose services were enlisted during the week of the American Psychiatric Association's annual convention in St. Louis. Advantage was thus taken of the opportunity to interview at one time many hospital executives who were in attendance at the convention. In this way numerous personal contacts were made, with a minimum of travel. In addition, institutions in various parts of the country were visited. For the rest, detailed questionnaires were employed to secure the desired information. These were mailed in each instance to the hospital superintendent, with a covering letter requesting his personal coöperation. On account of illness Dr. Fitzpatrick was obliged to withdraw from the assignment and in December, 1936, was succeeded by Dr. Winfred Overholser, late Commissioner of Mental Diseases of Massachusetts, who completed the survey. (Dr. Overholser has since been appointed Superintendent of St. Elizabeths Hospital, Washington, D. C.).

Through questionnaires, personal interviews and visits, information was secured in reference to 224 public institutions out of a total of 273. In the accompanying table there

SUMMARY OF RETURNS

Regional Areas	ALL QUESTIONNAIRES			STATE HOSPITALS		
	Sent	Returned	Percentage Returned	Number of State Hospitals in Region	State Hospital Questionnaires Returned and Analyzed	Percentage
New England.	29	24	82.8	21	13	61.9
Middle Atlantic.	57	50	87.7	31	28	90.3
East No. Central	52	49	94.2	35	29	82.9
West No. Central	35	31	88.6	24	17	70.8
South Atlantic.	31	24	77.4	19	14	73.7
East So. Central	16	8	50.0	10	5	50.0
West So. Central	20	12	60.0	11	8	72.7
Mountain.	17	13	76.5	9	6	66.7
Pacific.	16	13	81.3	11	7	63.6
Total.	273	224*	82.1	171	127	74.3

* Ten returned questionnaires did not give sufficient information to warrant their inclusion in the analysis. The total number of hospitals on which the analysis was based was 214.

is presented a geographical distribution of the institutions approached and those responding, with a special tabulation for state hospitals.

Data were received from 82 per cent of all institutions to whom questionnaires were addressed and from 74 per cent of all the state hospitals in the country. The distribution by regional areas leads to the assumption that the data are fairly typical and offer a good cross section of information for the purpose of the study. On the supposition that any institution interested in research would reply and that, by the same token, only those without a serious interest in the problem would fail to do so, there is reason to believe that the greater proportion of the institutions engaging in research or manifesting a concern for it are represented in this coverage. An extended statistical analysis was made of the state hospitals, this group being by far the largest; while for the other groups certain general comments are offered. In this analysis assistance was given by Dr. Samuel W. Hamilton, Director, and Dr. Joseph Zubin, Statistician, of the Mental Hospital Survey Committee. Mr. Paul Komora, Associate Secretary, and other members of the National Committee's staff also collaborated in the work.

The study was organized to secure data on all aspects of the hospital situation having a material bearing on research activities or potentialities. Each hospital was appraised in reference to nineteen items that might furnish the basis for an estimate of the degree of suitability of the institution as a center for investigatory work. On the assumption that an appropriate hospital setting for research involves adequate staffing, facilities and arrangements for sound clinical work, together with an affiliation with a medical school or scientific center, there were included among the nineteen items of inquiry such matters as the ratio of medical and nursing personnel to patients, provisions for special therapies, out-patient and social services, professional training programs, medical library, laboratories, contact with a university center, and staff members serving on medical school faculties.

SUMMARY OF FINDINGS

The following facts and trends were revealed through the survey:

(1) Twenty of the 273 public institutions can be designated as research centers because of the character and quality of their investigatory work, the caliber of their personnel and the resources at their disposal for scientific studies. Descriptive notes relating to these hospitals are presented in Section III of this report.

(2) In addition to these twenty centers there are thirty-two publicly supported hospitals that offer distinct possibilities for research work, judging by the advantages they enjoy in the way of basic facilities that lend themselves to investigative activities. These institutions have made creditable arrangements for the care and treatment of patients and, although little or no research is being conducted, there are indications that, with encouragement and some financial assistance, promising developments might be expected.

(3) Some 150 of the 1,700 staff physicians in the public mental institutions of the country show a marked interest in and ability for investigative work.

(4) At the present time 219 research projects in state hospitals are under way or definitely planned. The investigations can be grouped under such a wide range of headings as clinical, therapeutic, biochemical, neuroanatomical, neurophysiological, constitutional, hereditary, endocrine, statistical, and psychiatric aspects of general medicine.

(5) Research interest is most marked in the Middle Atlantic, New England and East North Central States.

(6) Present conditions are not favorable for the prosecution of research in 80 per cent of the institutions covered by this study.

(7) It is estimated that not more than two or three

million dollars are expended annually for psychiatric research in the United States and that, of this amount, more than half is derived from foundations, individuals and private agencies.

(8) A large majority of hospital superintendents who were queried in the survey were in favor of state hospital participation in research. But in answer to the question, "Should research undertakings in your State be centralized in one research institute?" half of the men answered in the affirmative and half in the negative.

(9) There is unanimity among hospital superintendents concerning the desirability of close linkage between mental hospitals and medical schools wherever such liaison is feasible.

(10) Superintendents stated that the chief deterrents to the prosecution of research in mental hospitals are inadequate staffs, remuneration insufficient to attract the best men, difficulty in securing facilities and lack of funds for investigatory purposes.

(11) All superintendents agreed that research activities in hospitals tended to quicken the scientific interest of the staff, thereby improving the care and treatment of patients.

(12) In twenty-one hospitals, the research facilities were being used by outside groups.

(13) In the federal hospitals for the mentally ill, under the jurisdiction of the Veterans' Administration, the policy is favorable to the prosecution of research.

(14) Although there is a vast field for research in mental deficiency and convulsive disorders, there is a dearth of interest in investigative work in many of the institutions devoting attention to these conditions.

(15) The survey has furnished tangible evidence to indicate that a creditable beginning has been made in the development of research in public institutions, that there is a genuine interest on the part of hospital superintendents in the extension of investigatory work, that many worthwhile developments might be fostered with modest encour-

agement and financial support, and that the time is ripe for the inclusion of psychiatric research as an integral part of public policy in a number of states that hitherto have devoted little attention to this matter.

SUGGESTED MEASURES TO FACILITATE PROGRESS

As a result of this orientation survey of research in publicly supported hospitals of the United States, there have been revealed valuable leads for further endeavor. Those who have been connected with the study are convinced that a signal contribution might be made in placing mental hygiene and psychiatric research on a firmer and more productive basis in this country, if a capable group of scientists, having access to research funds, could devote attention during the next few years to such issues as the following: strengthening the existing twenty research centers to facilitate the training of research personnel for other hospitals; collaboration with the thirty-two potential centers to foster investigatory work; securing greater recognition for psychiatric research as a matter of public policy in the more progressive States; fostering closer affiliations between mental hospitals and medical schools; and recruiting promising young scientists for research activities in the field of psychiatry. A brief discussion of these issues follows.

The twenty hospitals that are actively engaged in research activities are in a position to contribute to the extension of investigatory work in other hospitals through the training of research personnel. And, while these institutions are today helpful in this regard, greater assistance might be effected through a suitably administered fellowship program, whereby promising men could be loaned and attached to these centers for training, and later placed in strategic posts. There is little doubt that suitable men would be welcomed by these various centers because, during the survey, requests were received for assistance in the furtherance of projects demanding additional workers.

In reference to the thirty-two institutions wherein arrangements seem to be suitable for research, there is provided an opportunity to convert at least some of these potential centers into active centers. Progress might be made in this direction by making contacts with the superintendents and governing bodies of these hospitals and by suggesting that, in the appointment of new staff members, preference be given to at least one candidate with research interests and suitable scientific training. Questions relating to flexibility of time-table and appropriate remuneration would also be canvassed.

As has been indicated in this report, there are a number of progressive States where research could be fostered if it became duly recognized as an essential activity in a well-rounded mental hygiene program. And it would seem that some States, if granted encouragement by a representative group of scientists, might take forward steps in this respect.

There is a growing realization among hospital psychiatrists of the advantages that result in the furtherance of research through close affiliation with medical schools and other scientific institutions. And now that psychiatry is receiving more and more attention by those engaged in medical education, there is a greater tendency to look to mental hospitals for collaboration. This movement for coöperative effort might be fostered by extending throughout the country arrangements similar to those recently initiated in Illinois, where a joint committee composed of representatives of the hospitals and medical schools of the State is engaged in developing programs to effect liaison.

The extension of research will be dependent, in large measure, upon the availability of men with eager and inquiring minds who possess the qualifications for exploratory endeavor. Up to the present time psychiatry has not been as fortunate as some other fields of medicine in recruiting the ablest individuals who might be expected to extend knowledge in this field. In an attempt to improve this situation, much might be gained by making contacts with recent graduates in medicine whose records would indicate promising careers in psychiatric research.

PART II

INTERPRETATION OF FINDINGS WITH REFERENCE TO STATE HOSPITALS

Part II

Interpretation of Findings with Special Reference to State Hospitals

STATE HOSPITALS

IT is interesting to examine more closely the situation with reference to the state hospital group, with which we must necessarily identify our study in the main, since these institutions care for the bulk of hospitalized mental cases and constitute the backbone of public treatment facilities for the mentally ill. More than 80 per cent of all patients in all the mental institutions of the country, public and private, are in state hospitals. An appraisal of their status, by weighing the various elements that are pertinent for research, seemed to be indicated, and was consummated in connection with 127 state hospitals. For the purposes of the study, the States were grouped into nine regional areas, in accordance with the standard distribution employed in the United States census statistics, namely: New England, Middle Atlantic, East North Central, East South Central, South Atlantic, West North Central, West South Central, Mountain, and Pacific States. (See Appendix "B".)

Hospital Ratings

An attempt was made to evaluate the hospitals in terms of basic situational factors, and a statistical method of rating was used for purposes of comparison. (See Section IV.) In the plan adopted each hospital was appraised in reference to 19 specific items. To illustrate: One of the items related to the type of clinical director. Institutions without clinical directors were given a rating of 0; those in which the superintendent served in this capacity were given a rating of 1; where a regular staff physician served, a rating of 2; and where a special clinical director was in charge, a rating of 3. The maximum number of points possible in this scoring for all the items was 66. Details of the rating and code are set forth in Section IV and Appendix "A".

The medians of these scores were computed for each group of States for each item, though all the details are not included, as the significance of some of the items taken alone is not great. Taken together, however, they serve as a valuable indicator of a hospital's capacity for investigative work.

One of the items receiving attention was the ratio of physicians to patients because, among other things, it seemed important from the point of view of time available for research work. The standard ratio advocated by the American Psychiatric Association is one physician to 150 patients. Most of the state hospitals fell short of this requirement, and only seven hospitals were found to better this ratio: three in New York and one each in Delaware, Massachusetts, Michigan, and Wisconsin.

The percentage of overcrowding, while an important influencing factor, was left out of the rating entirely, because the basis for estimating bed capacities varies so from State to State that the available figures for overcrowding are practically valueless. It was found that some of the institutions reporting themselves as not overcrowded appeared to be poor in all other facilities, indicating that their self-appraisal regarding capacity was probably inaccurate. On the other hand, it was found that some of the more serious overcrowding reported in the study existed in institutions otherwise rating high.

The ratings are valid only in presenting a rough picture of the soil in which a fertile researcher might reasonably be expected to flourish. There are left out of account the qualifications of the men who are conducting or planning research activities, as this factor can be only subjectively measured. But while in investigatory work "the man, like the play, is the thing," nevertheless, the setting for research is of sufficient significance to warrant the canvass that has been made.

Ratings in Reference to Regional Distribution

Taking the hospitals by regional groupings, we find, according to basic factors, the following distribution of ratings for the country. While the detailed ratings by specific items, as pointed out, are of doubtful value when taken separately, in combination they present something of a picture of the existing possibilities and potentialities for research activity in state hospitals. Table IV, in Section IV, gives the regional distribution of total ratings for all the state hospitals surveyed. For convenience of interpretation, the ratings have been converted into percentages, computed on a basis of 100 instead of 66. For example, the rating for New England, 34.8, becomes 52.7 per cent. On a possible score of 100, we arrive at a general rating of 51.2 for the entire country. (See graph.) Following is the distribution of ratings by regional areas in descending order:

Middle Atlantic............ 63.3
New England.............. 52.7
East North Central.......... 49.5
West North Central.......... 46.1
Pacific................... 45.2
West South Central.......... 39.4
South Atlantic............. 35.6
Mountain................. 31.8
East South Central.......... 30.0

This analysis confirms what we know from previous observation and corresponds with what we would expect to find in one respect, namely, the primacy of the Middle Atlantic and New England States in clinical resources and the capacity for research activity which good clinical work connotes. These and the East North Central, West North Central and Pacific areas would seem to offer the most promising loci for investigative work, although here and there, in some of the Southern and Mountain States, interest and even activity in research are evident.

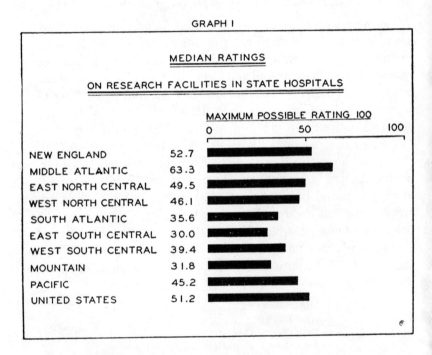

GRAPH I

MEDIAN RATINGS

ON RESEARCH FACILITIES IN STATE HOSPITALS

MAXIMUM POSSIBLE RATING 100

		0	50	100
NEW ENGLAND	52.7			
MIDDLE ATLANTIC	63.3			
EAST NORTH CENTRAL	49.5			
WEST NORTH CENTRAL	46.1			
SOUTH ATLANTIC	35.6			
EAST SOUTH CENTRAL	30.0			
WEST SOUTH CENTRAL	39.4			
MOUNTAIN	31.8			
PACIFIC	45.2			
UNITED STATES	51.2			

Types of Studies

At the present time, 219 research projects are under way or projected in state mental hospitals. A listing of the studies shows a considerable range and is indicative of the wide front upon which the problem of psychiatric research may be attacked, as well as a praiseworthy interest on the part of many workers. Using the classification employed

by the Index Medicus, these investigations fall under the
following heads:

Subject Classification	Number of Studies
Clinical, neurological and psychiatric	58
Clinical, convulsive disorders	6
Therapy (except those under next heading)	73
Psychotherapy, including medical psychology	11
Biochemistry and clinical laboratory	28
Neuroanatomy and neurophysiology	19
Constitutional, heredity, etc	7
Endocrine and vegetative nervous system	7
Administration and statistics	9
Psychiatric aspects of general medicine	1
Total	219

Supplementary Data

It was possible to secure from executive officers of 70
state hospitals their judgments and opinions on a number
of important matters that are relevant to research. And
there follows an epitomization of some of the reactions
gleaned in this way.

In reply to the query "Should research undertakings
in your state be centralized in one research institute?" 25
superintendents answered in the affirmative and 26 in the
negative. In other words, there is, as we might expect, a
difference of opinion on this point. Significantly 19 did not
reply to this question. To the alternative question, "Or is
it advisable to develop a program wherein the various
mental hospitals participate?" 34 replied with a definite
"yes" and only 13 said frankly "no".

As to the desirability of close linkage between the mental
hospital and the medical school there is almost complete
unanimity, although the same unanimity does not exist
regarding the possibility of such relationship. This we
would expect, since many state hospitals are physically far
removed from medical teaching centers. In this connection
we find that a number of state hospitals are used by medical
schools as training centers, the students spending a stipu-

lated time in residence for psychiatric instruction. The advantages of this procedure, both for the students in training and for the stimulation of the staff physicians, are obvious.

Only about one-fourth of our informants were willing to express themselves as considering the opportunities for research "amply attractive." The most important drawbacks to research activity listed were: inadequacy of staff, with the resultant absorption of time in routine activities; insufficient pay to attract the right type of men for research; inadequate facilities; and lack of funds to devote to research.

On one point there was universal agreement, namely, the value of research activities in quickening the scientific interest of the staff and thereby improving the care and treatment of patients. Incidentally, it was found that in at least 21 instances the research facilities of the state hospitals were being used by outside groups.

Another important factor concerning which the institutions were queried was the attitude toward research on the part of governing bodies (state departments, boards of control, boards of trustees, etc.). This was described as "good" in 25 cases, "neutral" in 24, and "unfavorable" in 2. Nineteen did not answer this question.

The absence of available funds was pointed out in 29 instances, described as "limited" in 15, and as having no particular limit in 8. As to time available for research work, 15 reported full time, 25 part time, 8 none, and 22 were silent on this point.

The training and experience of staff members in research was reported as "good" in 31 instances, "fair" in 5, and "poor" in 6. Sixty hospitals reported technicians, and 46 a full-time pathologist. Training schools for nurses were reported in 21 hospitals.

To sum up, it would appear from these inquiries that central planning of research, with participation by individual hospitals, is considered helpful; that close linkage of the medical school and mental hospital is desirable; and that inducements should be offered in order to attract and hold promising research workers, particularly in the form of better salaries and freer time for investigative activities.

TEACHING HOSPITALS

The psychopathic hospitals, so called, though few in number and not of great size, care for a large number of patients yearly on a short term basis, and are significant as research centers. A notable example is the New York Psychiatric Institute and Hospital in New York City, which is devoted primarily to research, at an annual expense of $500,000. There is a large and capable staff, selected on the basis of research ability and aptitude. Some forty distinct research projects are being conducted at present at this center. Another outstanding institution, also located in New York City, is Bellevue Psychiatric Hospital, where a well-developed research program is being carried on, in spite of great burdens imposed by a tremendous admission rate (25,000 patients per year), with twenty-five projects now under way.

Other important and active centers of this type are: Boston Psychopathic Hospital, Boston, Mass.; State Psychopathic Hospital, Ann Arbor, Mich.; Colorado Psychopathic Hospital, Denver, Colo.; Wisconsin Psychiatric Institute, Madison, Wis.; and the State Psychopathic Hospital, Iowa City, Ia.

Among special research institutions, though not strictly speaking psychopathic hospitals, should be mentioned the Illinois Research Hospital and the Institute for Juvenile Research, both in Chicago. The total number of psychopathic hospitals for which data were obtained was 11.

FEDERAL HOSPITALS

The Federal Government conducts a number of mental hospitals. Outstanding among them is St. Elizabeths Hospital in Washington, D. C. Under the administration of

the late Dr. William A. White, several significant researches—laboratory, clinical and psychological—were
initiated at this institution and are still in progress under
the supervision of the present Superintendent, Dr. Winfred Overholser. The largest group of federal hospitals
for the mentally ill are those under the Veterans' Administration, and a research program is under way in these
institutions, notably at Northport, New York. Several
studies have been made at other veterans' hospitals, especially in Palo Alto, California; Lyons, New Jersey; and
Tuskegee, Alabama. The policy of the Veterans' Administration is distinctly one of encouragement of research
activities. Information was received regarding 23 hospitals in this group. The physical facilities and arrangements and the ratio of physicians and nurses to patients
are excellent, and the soil in general is fertile for research
in these institutions.

INSTITUTIONS FOR THE FEEBLEMINDED AND EPILEPTICS

There are 72 public institutions for the feebleminded and
epileptic and 10 for the care of epileptics alone with a total
patient population exceeding 90,000. While it was impossible to make a detailed study of these institutions, the fact
was elicited that research was not receiving the attention
it deserves. This statement does not apply to Letchworth
Village, New York, or the Wrentham State School, Massachusetts, and a number of other training centers for mental
defectives. Studies in the field of convulsive disorders
are in progress at the following institutions: State Village
for Epileptics, Skillman, New Jersey; Monson State Hospital, Monson, Massachusetts; Craig Colony for Epileptics,
Sonyea, New York; and the Boston City Hospital, Boston,
Massachusetts. Interest is also in evidence in such places
as the Newark State School, Newark, New York, and in
some of the Pennsylvania institutions, but it is obvious that
much more can and should be done in the domains of
mental deficiency and convulsive disorders.

PART III

DESCRIPTION OF LEADING RESEARCH CENTERS

Part III

Description of Twenty Leading Research Centers

T HERE are submitted in this section brief outlines of the clinical, teaching and research arrangements in the tax-supported institutions, covered by this survey, that are furnishing leadership in the investigatory field. The following institutions are described:

Colorado	Colorado Psychopathic Hospital, Denver
District of Columbia	St. Elizabeths Hospital, Washington
Illinois	Elgin State Hospital, Elgin Illinois Psychiatric Institute, Chicago Institute for Juvenile Research, Chicago
Indiana	Central State Hospital, Indianapolis
Iowa	Iowa State Psychopathic Hospital, Iowa City
Maryland	Spring Grove State Hospital, Catonsville
Massachusetts	Boston Psychopathic Hospital, Boston Boston State Hospital, Boston Worcester State Hospital, Worcester Wrentham State School, Wrentham
Michigan	Neuropsychiatric Institute, Ann Arbor Wayne County Training School, Northville Ypsilanti State Hoscpital, Ypsilanti
New York	Bellevue Psychiatric Hospital, New York City Letchworth Village, Thiells State Psychiatric Institute, New York City
Ohio	Columbus State Hospital, Columbus
Wisconsin	Wisconsin Psychiatric Institute, Madison

COLORADO PSYCHOPATHIC HOSPITAL
Denver, Colorado

The Colorado Psychopathic Hospital is one of the outstanding psychiatric centers of the country. The institution was founded by the people for the treatment of individuals who are experiencing acute or incipient types of personality disorders. The hospital serves the State in three ways. First, through the clinical facilities of the hospital; second, through the follow-up care which is carried on in the out-patient department; and finally, through the various community clinics which are being maintained at strategic points throughout the State. The staff is composed of fifteen members (four senior men, seven Commonwealth Fund fellows, one director of the Psychiatric Liaison Department, and three United States Public Health Service men). The director is professor of psychiatry at the University of Colorado and is affiliated with the Summer School and Law School of the University of Denver.

The Colorado Psychopathic Hospital is affiliated with the University of Colorado and has a very extensive teaching program which deals with both undergraduates and graduates. The hospital staff gives 150 hours of psychiatry to the University of Colorado School of Medicine, and 30 hours of psychiatry to the School of Nursing. This instruction in psychiatry includes not only lectures but demonstrations, clinical clerkships, training in out-patient department, and ward work. Since the establishment of the Commonwealth Fund fellowships in 1928, twenty-four physicians have completed their training and the majority have acquired teaching positions in universities throughout the country. Others have entered the mental hygiene movement, child guidance clinics, or important positions in either state or private hospitals. The United States Public Health Service has assigned five men to the hospital for psychiatric training. Two of these men have been assigned to important posts in the mental hygiene division of the United States Public Health Service; three are still in training.

A recent teaching project has been the exchange of Fellowship men with physicians on the staff of the Colorado State Hospital. Ward rounds held twice weekly and a weekly conference and seminar provide opportunity for study and discussion in addition to that obtained in the case work. The teaching program also includes summer school classes, lectures and demonstrations to the University of Denver School of Law, and the School of Social Work, as well as several extension classes sponsored by the University of Colorado.

Further educational activities of the hospital include annual conferences on recent advances in psychiatry with state hospital superintendents of the Rocky Mountain Region, monthly bulletins on some timely psychiatric subject addressed to the medical profession, and addresses on mental hygiene, child guidance and other topics to other professional and lay groups in the community.

The Colorado Psychopathic Hospital out-patient department, or Clinic, is a member of the Council of Social Agencies of Denver, and coöperates with doctors, schools, courts and other agencies, which refer cases for treatment and study.

A grant by the Rockefeller Foundation has made possible the establishment of a Psychiatric Liaison Department in the Colorado General Hospital. The clinical and educational program of this department has resulted in a closer union between medicine and psychiatry.

The research projects of the hospital are varied and multiple. Each member of the staff is encouraged to follow some original investigation, and certain members show outstanding abilities along this line. One of the more important studies is that with syphilis of the central nervous system which has been carried on since 1925. The therapeutic effect of malaria followed by specific chemotherapy is being investigated through this study. Prognostic studies are likewise being carried out in this group. With respect to syphilis of the central nervous system, a comparative study is now being made between malarial-treated paretics and those who are receiving artificial pyretotherapy (Kettering Hypertherm). Recently the hospital was made a member of the group studying the non-specific treatment of neurosyphilis under the direction of the United States Public Health Service.

With respect to fever therapy interesting studies are being made upon Sydenham's chorea, central nervous system syphilis, the arthritides, gonorrhea and certain degenerative diseases of the central nervous system. Special attention is being directed to the nature of the deliria experienced by the fever patients. In addition, certain biochemical aspects of some of these problems are being studied.

As in other clinics throughout the country, research is being centered upon the schizophrenic problem. Prognostic studies and the use of insulin in schizophrenia are in progress. Studies consisting of detailed mental examinations and the Rorschach test are being utilized in the study of schizophrenics treated with insulin. By this means it is hoped that a better understanding can be reached concerning the qualitative type of remission in these patients. Special biochemical studies are being conducted during the hypoglycemic therapy of the schizophrenic.

The Rorschach test itself is being given a place of importance in the research program. Its use as a special method of studying the personality is noteworthy.

Other important major projects include causal and therapeutic significance of the Vitamin B complex in chronic alcoholics; a special study of alcoholism with reference to quantitative blood and urine studies and their relation to motor accidents; the quantitative determination of estrogens in normal women and those mentally ill; a study of juvenile delinquency; the use of the association motor in the psychoneuroses; and encephalography.

A total budget for the hospital of $175,000 per year allows very little for research *per se*. The rather extensive research program outlined above is made possible only through the lively interest and coöperation of all members of the staff. The exact amount spent for research would be difficult to estimate. Certainly, additional funds are needed for further studies into the problems of schizo-phrenia, alcoholism and electro-encephalography.

ST. ELIZABETHS HOSPITAL
Washington, D. C.

St. Elizabeths is a federal institution under the Department of the Interior, and is devoted to the treatment of mental patients from the District of Columbia and members and former members of the military and naval services and other beneficiaries of the Government. It is the largest of all the federal mental hospitals and has long been one of the foremost psychiatric centers of the country, with an outstanding record of scientific achievement. It is also one of the most completely equipped, having besides its well-appointed psychiatric and neurological services, a department of medicine and surgery which includes in its subdivisions the following clinics: gynecology, urology, syphilology, ophthalmology, otolaryngology, dermatology, physiotherapy, radiology, dentistry, and special facilities for tuberculosis and contagious diseases. These services are rounded out by well-equipped facilities for physical and occupational therapy, social services, a dietetic service, clinical and pathological laboratories, and a nursing school. It does not conduct an out-patient service. It has a well-stocked medical library of over 15,000 volumes.

St. Elizabeths is also a leading training center. It is affiliated with George Washington University Medical School, Howard University School of Medicine and the Naval Medical School, and courses in psychiatry and related subjects are given to other institutions also, such as the University of Maryland. A number of its staff members are on the faculties of one or more of these institutions. It conducts a regular three-year course in its nursing school, as well as post-graduate courses, and receives affiliate nurses from four local hospitals. Its social service department also trains students, both from its own and other organizations in the district. It has a large junior medical staff and trains at least eight internes a year. It has a first-rate laboratory housed in a large building of its own, where up to 65 per cent of deaths are autopsied.

The research interests of the staff are extensive and varied and original work has been done in several fields. Subjects of study deal with the following, among others: malaria and diathermy treatment of dementia paralytica; disorders of muscle tone and their localizing significance; oxycephaly; psychogenetics of crime and suicide; drug therapy; Berger rhythm waves; and metabolism. Psychological research has been undertaken on deterioration in dementia praecox. This study covers psychological material which has been accumulated over a period of fifteen years in the hospital, in the hope of learning more about the intellectual functions in disease types, as an aid to early diagnosis and other procedures.

The amount of money spent on research work is difficult to estimate, but the total annual allotment, including salaries, for the laboratory during 1937 and 1938 is $37,500.

ELGIN STATE HOSPITAL
Elgin, Illinois

Elgin State Hospital has had an active research program for several years. It is in close contact with local educational centers, six of its staff members teaching in the Chicago medical schools, and has good training facilities. Between six and eight internes a year are taken on at the hospital for six-months' training periods. Regular courses are conducted, with nine or ten weekly clinical conferences. It has a limited staff of occupational therapists. Its outpatient and social services are likewise limited. Much teaching is carried on by giving ward talks and clinical lectures to various groups of students from colleges in the northern part of the state. The hospital conducted a nursing school for many years, but discontinued it in accordance with the policy of the Department of Public Welfare to reduce the number of training schools in the State.

It has a good laboratory, which functions as a central state laboratory for Illinois charitable institutions, and its facilities are available to all state mental hospitals. A large number of autopsies are performed.

Eight of its staff members have research interests, and several have training and experience in special fields, such as the physical sciences, neuropathology, and chemistry. A full-time psychologist is constantly doing research as well as routine work in her special line. There is a provision in the statutes that five per cent of the State's budget for all state hospitals can be used for investigative work but it has never been utilized in practice—no part of this sum ever having been apportioned to an individual state hospital—and most of the research work is done inter-currently with other activities.

The research facilities of the hospital are also used by outside specialists. Elgin's progressive-minded superintendent emphasizes the fact that the hospital is open ''as a workshop, to psychiatrists, psychologists and sociologists who have problems in the working out of which the study of cases or case records may be of assistance.'' Besides its own library, the hospital has the use of reference facilities in the local universities.

Considerable work has been done in fever therapy on patients suffering from syphilis, dementia praecox and, to some extent, on the manic-depressive psychoses. Prolonged sleep therapy was tried for a time but discontinued pending the establishment of safer and more adequate treatment conditions for this procedure. Experiments have also been undertaken in insulin therapy. Forty patients are now under treatment with insulin and eighty with metrazol. A physiological chemist has just been employed to collaborate with the hospital's neuropathologist and clinicians in an investigation of the various problems connected with these treatments. A well equipped biochemical laboratory is being developed.

The "Elgin Papers" (second volume) just published by the hospital and distributed widely in and out of the State, reflect the varied scope of its research activities. They report investigations of such problems as alcoholism and the psychoses, heat regulation in dementia praecox, Huntington's chorea, hematoporphyrin treatment of severe depressions, suicide, endocrinopathies and psychoses, dieto-therapy in dementia praecox, and the effect of sodium amytal on the oxygen consumption rate in the psychoses. Work is in progress also on reactions to pitressin in dementia praecox, benzedrine in post-encephalitis and dementia praecox, snake venom and rabies therapy in epilepsy, cardiosol as a test for latent epilepsy, group psychotherapy, and other therapeutic approaches. Funds are needed to enable the hospital to extend its investigations of the organic and functional aspects and their interrelations in schizophrenia, a problem in which it is especially interested at this time.

ILLINOIS PSYCHIATRIC INSTITUTE
Chicago, Illinois

The Illinois Psychiatric Institute is a part of the Research and Educational Hospitals which are operated jointly by the State Department of Public Welfare and the Medical College of the University of Illinois.

The clinical facilities include an out-patient department and sixty beds for psychotic patients. The staff includes a part-time director, four full-time psychiatrists and four part-time psychiatrists. There are also three full-time residents provided by the University and at the present time there are three full-time fellows provided by the Department of Public Welfare and a prospect of one additional fellow.

There are 13 graduate nurses, 18 attendants, an occupational therapy supervisor, and a social worker, and the personnel of the other units of this medical center are available for consultations on problems relating to the various branches of medicine. Occupational therapy is administered to about 50 per cent of the Institute's patients. About 100 cases are under its social service supervision annually.

The Institute has the services of a pathologist and technician, in addition to a small local laboratory. The pathological work is done in connection with the department of neurology, which is now separate from that of psychiatry, and a part-time histologist is provided by the Department of Public Welfare. In addition the Institute has the services of a full-time professor of physiology made possible through a grant from the Rockefeller Foundation to which reference will be made below. Assistance in psychologic testing is secured through the Institute for Juvenile Research which is maintained by the Department of Public Welfare on the same campus. There is also a part-time psychologist provided through the W.P.A. And there are two full-time psychiatric social workers.

Four internes are trained each year by the seminar method, with opportunities for experience in regular clinical activities, out-patient services, laboratory work, and clinical research. A system of undergraduate teaching has been introduced with the aid of the grant from the Rockefeller Foundation. This system has for its main objective a closer integration between psychiatry and physiology. Psychiatric instruction is being given during the first and second years interlocking with appropriate facilities for physiologic teaching, and some of the physiologic work has been advanced to the third year. Psychiatric instruction is given during the third year on the medical wards and students in the senior year, in addition to receiving didactic instruction, serve for two weeks in the out-patient department and one week of clerkship in the psychiatric wards. This development is considered as a research project.

Graduate instruction is being given to residents and fellows planned to meet the requirements of the American Board of Psychiatry and Neurology. All these positions are for three years.

The Institute is adequately set up for research purposes and practically all staff members are engaged in some research project. A five-year program of research is now nearing completion. A systematic investigation of a clinical study of patients by means of measurable responses to routine situations for specially devised situations has been carried on for the past two years. It seems probable that some material will be ready for publication within a short time.

During this past year intensive study and development of therapy by the use of the various forms of shock treatment in certain combinations have been under way and some of the results are ready for publication. In addition certain work is being carried on in certain special fields such as the study of the electric skin resistance under various conditions; studies of the capillaries of the skin and various problems in connection with the use of insulin and metrazol of a physiologic nature.

Money has been made available by the General Assembly of Illinois for the erection of a Neuropsychiatric Institute which will permit the training of many more graduate students and a large increase in the equipment especially for physiological research in this field. It is expected that the Institute will be fully equipped from a physical point of view. The only point that remains for real concern in this connection is that of adequate appropriation for salaries and operation. However, the Department of Public Welfare has expressed itself as anxious to coöperate in this direction as fully as may be possible.

The Institute will include both neurologic and psychiatric divisions and will be the center of psychiatric teaching in the College of Medicine. It is planned to include facilities also in the Institute for teaching and research to be carried on by each of the four medical schools in the city of Chicago.

The department of psychiatry and the College of Medicine are providing instruction and supervision of continuous research for the state hospitals in the northern part of the State.

Regular courses of instruction are given to state hospital physicians who are assigned for duty to the Institute for that purpose by the Department of Public Welfare.

A well-stocked library, including from fifteen to twenty current journals, is extensively used. In addition, the ample reference facilities of the university library are available to the Institute.

Institute for Juvenile Research
Chicago, Illinois

This is a state-supported institution for the study and treatment of behavior problems in children, organized in 1909 as the Juvenile Psychopathic Institute under the Board of Cook County Commissioners by Dr. William Healy, following his notable five-year study of delinquents in the Chicago Juvenile Courts. In 1916 it was taken over by the Illinois Department of Public Welfare as the Institute for Juvenile Research as a part of the Division of the Criminologist. In addition to the clinic at headquarters in Chicago, the Institute conducts community and branch clinics in various parts of the State; maintains a training center for psychiatrists, psychologists, psychiatric social workers, and research sociologists; and conducts researches in various fields related to the treatment and prevention of delinquency and personality disorders.

The headquarters clinic staff is divided into two groups, the smaller group offering diagnostic and consultative service; the larger group, comprising the bulk of the Institute staff, devoting itself to the treatment of cases selected by the first group from the clinical material which comes under its survey. The medical personnel includes seven experienced full-time psychiatrists, and four fellows in psychiatry, and there is a staff of eight psychiatric social workers, and nine full-time psychologists. There are three social workers who have specialized in recreation problems; and other personnel participate from time to time, for example, a remedial reading worker and research psychologists engaged on special projects.

About 1,500 patients pass through the clinic yearly, mostly children under 14 years of age. The ratio of boys to girls is about two to one, and there are about two cases referred from individuals, schools, and similar sources to every three from social case work organizations. About a fifth of the incoming cases are sent by the courts. Of these some 45 per cent are diagnostic and advisory cases, 35 per cent are coöperative cases, and 20 per cent are selected for intensive psychiatric and social treatment.

Under the Institute's scheme of organization there is a psychiatric service; a psychological service for intelligence measurements and special diagnostic tests, vocational and educational counsel; a social service and a recreation service. Medical examinations are given by psychiatrists when indicated. The community clinic program of the Institute, in operation for the past fifteen years, has as its purpose the development of local community resources so that each community may be equipped to meet its own problems of child guidance. In addition to the conduct of established community clinics, the Institute also extends its services to other parts of the State, in terms of complete and partial examinations of problem children.

Noteworthy among the Institute's community activities is the Chicago Area Project, which represents an attempt to discover a procedure for the more effective treatment and prevention of delinquency in certain of the deteriorated areas in the city of Chicago. Programs are being carried on in three such communities. The first of these was initiated in 1932.

In this project an attempt is being made to develop a

community-wide activities program for all of the children residing in each of the areas. The essential feature of the project is the emphasis which is placed upon the participation of the parents and other local residents in planning and operating every phase of the program. A council of local residents has been organized in each of the three areas. These local groups not only assist in formulating the policies of the program, but they seek to utilize in a coördinated manner all of the facilities available in all of the institutions and agencies in the local community. It is assumed that by stimulating the local community to act in its own behalf new values may be introduced which will provide a more constructive social environment for the children.

Detailed records are being kept of all cases of school truants, juvenile delinquents, and adult criminals to determine the effectiveness of the program as applied to the treatment and prevention of delinquency.

Finally, there are the medical, psychological, and social service research aspects of the Institute's program, and its comprehensive training and educational activities. In addition to examining children and assuming responsibility for the training of students, the Institute further influences community thinking through courses in medical and social work schools and by single lectures and short series of lectures. The teaching material is presented through the medium of its case records.

In connection with its professional training program, the Institute maintains intimate contact with several university teaching centers, among them the University of Illinois, Rush Medical College, Northwestern University and Loyola University. During the autumn and winter of 1936, for example, a course in the management of children's behavior problems was offered to physicians for the third time. The course was conducted under the auspices of the Illinois University College of Medicine by the Institute

Director and the Institute pediatrician. Several members of the Institute staff serve on college faculties.

The Institute trains four psychiatric fellows each year, under the seminar and fellowship type of teaching and supervision. It also gives training to students in clinical psychology, who come from the various universities after having completed at least one semester of graduate work in psychology in the University, and spend at least six months at the Institute doing psychological work. Another activity of the department of psychology is the training of teachers and tutors in the technique of giving remedial instruction in reading. Students of social work also come to the Institute for field work.

Three members of the present psychiatric staff are participating in the research program of the Chicago Institute for Psychoanalysis. Since 1936 there has been in process a research project on play room methods for the individual, direct treatment of neurotic children. Two research projects with a medical orientation may be particularly mentioned. One is concerned with the relation of congenital syphilis to children's behavior problems, in an attempt to differentiate more adequately certain types of behavior which are the results of cerebral syphilis and other types related to family disorganization; the other is a study of the role of heart disease in the production of children's behavior problems.

Researches by the department of psychology include statistical studies of delinquency (particularly the measurement of intelligence of children in a delinquency area); an investigation of the relative stability of intelligence quotients at various age levels; the development and standardization of non-verbal studies; and studies of the psychogalvanic reflex and other problems in physiological psychology.

The social service department has studied the effects of the depression on family life, and a statistical study of intake is in progress, covering all children examined by the

Institute, with particular reference to the problems for which they were referred, sources from which referred, social background and other factors.

CENTRAL STATE HOSPITAL
Indianapolis, Indiana

The Central State Hospital is the only one of the Indiana state hospitals active in research work. It has one of the largest and best equipped neuropathological laboratories in the country for research in mental diseases. It is closely affiliated with the University Hospitals of Indiana University, and serves as a teaching center in psychiatry for Indiana University School of Medicine. The superintendent is professor of psychiatry and head of the department of nervous and mental diseases of the Medical School, and the director of laboratories is clinical professor of psychiatry. There is a training program for residents in psychiatry. There is, however, no training school for mental nurses and no social service connected with the hospital. Since the nearby Indiana University Hospitals operate a psychiatric out-patient department which is directed by a staff member of the institution, the Central State Hospital does not operate an out-patient clinic of its own.

The facilities for special therapies are good, about 50 per cent of the patients being served by occupational therapy. The physical arrangements for laboratory work are excellent and well suited for research, a large two-story building being used for this purpose. Pathological work is extensive, with an autopsy rate of 50 per cent. Three technicians are employed in addition to the pathologist. There is a library of 1,200 volumes.

The laboratories were reorganized in 1931 after a visit by the director to all the important mental hospital laboratories in this country and abroad. There are no special funds, laboratory maintenance coming out of the institution's general operating expenses, and the cost of research has been small, since all investigative work is carried out as part of the routine work.

Extensive investigations have been carried on in the histopathology of the psychoses with subacute bacterial and chronic rheumatic endocarditis and on the histopathology of neurosyphilis. In collaboration with the U. S. Public Health Service, Washington, D. C., and with the Coöperative Clinical Group a comparative study is being made of the various types of non-specific therapy (malaria, artificial fever and other means) which are used at the present time in the treatment of general paralysis and other forms of neurosyphilis.

The director of the laboratories at this time is particularly interested in the frequency of chronic rheumatic brain disease found in dementia praecox patients. Another study deals with hypoplasia of the vascular system with particular emphasis on the size of the basilar artery in schizophrenic patients. Financial support (about $500 per annum) for special research into the somatic aspects of mental disease would be welcome.

IOWA STATE PSYCHOPATHIC HOSPITAL
Iowa City, Iowa

This is one of the leading western centers of psychiatric research, a teaching hospital attached to the State University of Iowa, with an active training program. Five members of the staff instruct classes at the medical school, and three conduct M.A. and Ph.D. theses investigations. The hospital trains two internes a year. It has a well-staffed out-patient and social service department. A feature of the institution is its speech correction clinic conducted by an expert in this field.

It has good research equipment, with special laboratories in chemistry, neuropathology, brain physiology and electrophysiology, a pathologist and two technicians. Autopsies at the medical college supply ample material for study. It has a well-stocked and much used library, including 300 medical journals. Over $10,000 was spent on books and journals during the past year.

There is an alert medical staff, and three of its nine physicians show rather outstanding characteristics from the research standpoint. The senior staff members all have special research interest, and the junior members are also stimulated to undertake research projects. Six of the staff have conducted investigations which have appeared in leading European and American journals. From one-half to three-quarters of their time is devoted to research, and special time is granted by the director for approved projects. Actually all teaching and clinical work done by the center has a bearing on research.

Special grants for research work have come from the Rockefeller Foundation, and state appropriations include a basic amount for this purpose. The state authorities are strongly favorable to the development of the institution's research activities. Liberal use of the institution's research facilities is made by graduate students from the University of Iowa.

Over 30 publications were produced by the staff during the past three years. Original work was done in the following fields: neurophysiological effects of intoxicating drugs; psychopathological effects of drugs affecting the vegetative system; histopathology of the brain; the blood and cerebrospinal fluid barrier; relationship between chloride content and blood cerebrospinal fluid bromide ratio; psychogenic motor disturbances; borderline psychoses; neurological aspects of stuttering; an action current study of handedness in relation to stuttering; effect of direct stimulation of brain and spinal cord on reflex time; and a study of retinal summation. Some limited but careful work on insulin therapy of schizophrenia is being done under control conditions. Funds are solicited for further work in electro-encephalography, and for studies in chronaxie.

Spring Grove State Hospital
Catonsville, Maryland

This is a typical state hospital serving the Baltimore metropolitan area, and includes a special division for the white criminal insane. It is the third oldest in the United States (founded in 1797), and the oldest of the Maryland state hospitals. At the same time it has one of the most modern buildings for the treatment of acute and curable cases and for those with physical ailments. It suffers, in common with Maryland's other state hospitals, in the inadequacy of its general treatment facilities—insufficiency of personnel, particularly of graduate nurses, and limited provisions for hydrotherapy, occupational therapy, and other special services. There is a training school for attendants but none for nurses. There is little extra-mural activity connected with the hospital, and no definite organization of out-patient clinics. Only one social worker is employed.

On the other hand, there is a definite and marked interest in scientific work, with a high percentage of autopsies in relation to deaths. The laboratory facilities are good and there is also the advantage of the hospital's close connections with the Phipps Psychiatric Clinic, with reference to pathological work. The facilities of Phipps are also available for training purposes. The hospital trains four internes each year, and, with improved resources, more could be done toward the development of an organized and systematic training program. Extensive use is made of the Johns Hopkins medical library.

Research activities have been undertaken in collaboration with the Phipps Clinic. Though only a limited time can be devoted to research work under present conditions, significant studies have been made in connection with insulin shock treatment, the results of which were reported at a recent meeting of the American Psychiatric Association. Were additional funds available, this work would be extended with a view to comparative investigations of insulin treatment with other forms of shock therapy, and the enlargement of the groups studied under these forms of treatment.

Plans are under way at the present time to secure funds to enable the hospital to employ another full-time physician and a sufficient number of nurses to carry groups of 10 to 15 patients continuously on intensive treatment, including the various forms of shock therapy. If these plans mature this hospital will become the center for the State for the treatment of selected cases from the other state hospitals. The primary problem is the matter of finances, and it is estimated that the research program contemplated will cost about $8,000.

BOSTON PSYCHOPATHIC HOSPITAL
Boston, Massachusetts

This is a representative institution of the university psychopathic hospital type established under public auspices for the intensive study and treatment of acute and incipient cases of mental disease, and for research and training purposes. It is one of the pioneers in its field, now in its twenty-fifth year, and exemplifies the early striving for psychiatric services that are in intimate contact with community life, in contrast to the more remote state hospital, and make for easier accessibility of the mentally sick to hospital care and earlier diagnosis and treatment.

Boston Psychopathic Hospital has three main functions: (1) that of a special health service to residents of metropolitan Boston and to patients from other districts of the Commonwealth who for various reasons may be referred to this hospital; (2) research into the nature and causes of mental disease, its prevention and treatment; (3) instruction of physicians and medical students in the principles and practice of psychiatry, and of psychologists, nurses, occupational workers, social workers in the special problems pertaining to this field of medicine. Its organization includes departments of occupational therapy, out-patient and social service, training of affiliated nurses, biochemical and psychological laboratories, and a department of therapeutic research.

Seven of the staff members are on college or university faculties. The director is professor of psychiatry at Harvard Medical School, and the lectures and clinical demonstrations for Harvard medical students are conducted at the hospital. There are eleven resident physicians and training and supervision consists of teaching and ward rounds, with staff conferences for one hour, five days a week. There is a library of over 6,000 books and 80 periodicals, on which a thousand dollars was spent in 1936. And there are well-equipped laboratories, including a variety of hyperpyrexia-producing apparatus.

A lively investigative spirit permeates the staff, its research interests being at present focused on schizophrenia, the physiological therapeutic aspects of hyperpyrexia in mental disorders, chemical studies pertaining to psychoses, especially the schizophrenias, blood studies of cases of delirium tremens, and hallucinations (organic aspect, audiometer, etc.). Special attention has been given to the syphilitic and alcoholic psychoses and various studies have been in progress in these fields.

Among researches of special note should be mentioned the statistical studies on schizophrenia which have been carried on at Boston Psychopathic Hospital since 1927. These are concerned not so much with the results of investigation as with the development of a more precise scientific methodology, in an attempt to sharpen the tools of research and to make investigative work more productive in all its aspects.

In contrast to these are the special studies of schizophrenia and the analysis of individual cases with these improved methods, to see whether the disorders of adaptation observed in patients may be due to some subtle disturbances of the fundamental chemical and physiological life processes. And at the other extreme from the detailed life processes dealt with in these investigations are the more complicated mental functions studied in the psychological laboratory. Here special problems have been taken up partly on account of their technical interest and partly on account of their immediate practical importance, such as the difficulties concerned with learning and the acquisition of skill, as well as with the difficulties of personal adjustment. Attention has for some time been concentrated in the laboratory on the special difficulties of reading which hamper many children.

A major project has been the comparative study of the results of tryparsamide treatment and malarial therapy in general paresis. In addition to the study of the effect of fever produced by malaria, studies have been made on the effect of fever induced by diathermy. Other studies in this field are concerned with the physiological effects of fever, with metabolism and velocity of blood flow in patients with therapeutic fever, both of the infectious disease and artificial types. Much original information concerning the acid-base balance of blood and brain, and concerning the part which the different elements of the body play in such adjustments has been obtained. The indicated interrelations have a rather broad biological significance. Likewise, much pioneer work has been done in the understanding of the regulation of respiration through these syphilitic studies. Through this work there has been gained a detailed and exact knowledge of physiological functions, which offers opportunity not only for comparison of the normal with the psychotic in regard to these functions, but also for the study of the control over these functions by the autonomic, endocrine, and humoral systems.

Extensive investigations of the effects of alcohol on the human organism, and of alcohol tolerance in relation to drinking habits, have also been under way. These include studies of the blood and spinal fluid alcohol, and of the factors which determine the blood alcohol curves, following intravenous and oral administration of alcohol; an experimental psychiatric study of acute alcoholic intoxication; and investigation of the effects of alcohol on reaction time and correlation of the blood alcohol level with these effects.

The hospital operates on a $200,000 budget, which does not meet all of its requirements for investigatory work. Funds are especially desired for the following projects: $12,000 for further schizophrenia studies; $1,500 for expanded work on the physiological therapeutic aspects of hyperpyrexia; and $5,000 for the extension studies pertaining to the psychoses, especially schizophrenia.

BOSTON STATE HOSPITAL
Boston, Massachusetts

This is a representative state hospital of the progressive type characteristic of the Massachusetts state hospital system. An indication of its dynamic and forward-looking attitude is its psychiatric clinic, established in 1933 to provide special treatment facilities of an intensive character for the more recoverable types of patients in a setting comparable to the specialized psychopathic hospital and conducive to better segregation of this group from the undifferentiated mass of long-term patients typically found in the average state hospital. In addition to its superior therapeutic arrangements, the hospital is in active contact with the community, through its first-rate out-patient and social services and its educational activities. Its professional training program includes lectures and clinical demonstrations for students from several institutions, among them Boston University School of Medicine, Middlesex College of Medicine and Surgery, Tufts Medical College, and Northeastern University. In addition to its own training school for mental nurses it gives psychiatric instruction to general nurses from surrounding hospitals. The hospital has a well developed pathological laboratory equipped for routine studies and for the prosecution of a comprehensive research program. It has a high autopsy rate. Its research division consists of a paid medical staff of seven workers and three unpaid medical workers, as well as paid technicians and a number of volunteer workers. Research activities come under three main headings, namely, human autonomic pharmacology, mineral studies, and clinical studies.

The scope of the studies in the first category is, fundamentally, to ascertain the effect of drugs of the autonomic series on human function and, if possible, to correlate them to the functions of the nervous system and those disorders which appear in the neuroses and psychoses. The subjects of study include the physiological effects of benzedrine and its relationship to other drugs affecting the autonomic nervous system; the effect of benzedrine sulfate on mood and fatigue in normal and in neurotic persons; the autonomic pharmacology of the gastric juices; the effect of benzedrine sulfate on the gall-bladder; the effect of mecholyl; the effect of cholinergic and adrenergic drugs on the eye; the synergism of prostigmin and mecholyl; and theories and results of autonomic drug administration. The work on esterase activity has been specially prosecuted in the last six months and some important results are now in press.

Studies in the second group deal with the mineral content of various cerebral lesions; experimental production of beri-beri in pigeons; and local anaphylactic lesions of the brain in guinea pigs. This work represents a relatively new departure in medicine, with its new technique of micro-incineration and the relatively new method of spectroscopic analysis of minerals. It is believed that important results have been obtained by these methods. The studies show, for example, that minerals are quantitatively dimin- ished in old age and in degenerative processes, and increased in youth and in actively growing tissue, such as tumors. The study of tumors has been especially striking in the mineral picture presented. Very signifi- cant differences have also been found in two types of feeblemindedness, one definitely representing a hyper- mineralization, and the other a mineral deficiency of strik- ing degree. These are the first real chemical differentia- tions of feeblemindedness. It has been shown, moreover, that essential differences between functionally active tis- sues are not only ascertainable but measurable. This work, it is believed, throws new and significant light on the nervous and bodily structures of man, both in health and disease.

The section on clinical studies has focused on the hereditary question in mental defect and mental disease, and did most of the work in the notable study of eugenical sterilization undertaken under the aegis of the American Neurological Association and recently published. The studies in this field are still in progress.

The research director has given especial attention to the structure of the neuroses, and this work is being actively prosecuted, especially in the relation of the neu- roses to the psychoses. It is believed that there is a funda- mental relationship between certain symptom groups in the neuroses and their evolution into the symptoms of the psychoses, especially the anxiety states.

The research division is financed in part by the State, in part by the Rockefeller Foundation and several small pri- vate funds. The total is, on the whole, not great and, it is felt, inadequate as compared to the scope of its investi- gations. About $27,000 is being spent annually on research activity, and additional funds of about $5,000 are now needed to develop the program.

Worcester State Hospital
Worcester, Massachusetts

Worcester State Hospital is one of the outstanding state hospitals of the country and conducts what are probably the most extensive research operations among the state hospitals of Massachusetts. It is superior, among other things, in the extent of its extra-institutional activities, having a strong out-patient and social service department, and devoting a considerable part of its energies and resources to professional and public education in mental health. In this respect it has set an example to the rest of the country, having led in the movement to break down the traditional isolation of state hospitals and to make them active community centers enlisting public interest and support comparable to that commonly accorded to general hospitals. In addition to its follow-up of paroled patients, it reaches out to those in danger of breaking down and, through its adult and child guidance clinic services, works for the prevention and control of mental and nervous disorders in its community.

Worcester State Hospital also engages in an active training program for the benefit of physicians, psychologists, social workers, educators, ministers and other professional workers concerned with the mentally ill, and has working affiliations or teaching contacts with a number of educational centers, among them Clark University, Tufts College, Boston University School of Medicine, Simmons College, and Smith College School of Social Work. It trains from two to four internes a year. Under its training plan, internes from Peter Bent Brigham Hospital serve four months in psychiatry, in addition to their internal medicine residencies. Internes are assigned to the admission wards for periods of six months, and under the supervision of the clinical director, are thoroughly drilled in the examination and study of patients in their various aspects: physical and mental status, neurological tests, personal and family histories, diagnosis, prognosis, presentation of cases at staff conferences, and follow-up treatment. It has an excellent medical library, of some 6,000 books and 120 periodicals, on which it spends about $1,500 annually.

The laboratory facilities are excellent, and while the physical plant is not entirely satisfactory, it is adequately equipped for routine and special activities. One criterion of the institution's investigative spirit and scientific bent is its high percentage of post-morten examinations, autopsies having been performed in over half of the number of deaths during the past year. Significant also is the fact that practically all the senior staff members have research interests, for which a comprehensive and varied research program, aided and abetted by the scientific outlook, encouragement and incentive of a progressive-minded administration, furnishes considerable outlet and scope and opportunity limited only by financial resources. Five of the members serve on college or university faculties.

Approximately $80,000 a year is now available for this institution's research activities, a major portion of which deal with dementia praecox, the most dominant type of hospitalized mental disease, numerically speaking, and the most obscure and perplexing of all problems that challenge psychiatric research and ingenuity. While special attention is being given to endocrinological factors, and a number of studies are geared on this level, the disease is being investigated from various angles, and parallel studies are in progress dealing with other forms and manifestations of mental disorder presenting related problems on the organic, physical, chemical, psychological and social levels. The broad approach to these problems is indicated in the wide range of projects under way or contemplated. Staff investigators are interested in such questions as the potentialities of insulin shock treatment and the development of other therapeutic methods for dementia praecox, biochemistry of the psychoses, endocrine therapy, treatment by pharmacological methods, physiological concomitants of mental disease, relationship of physical and mental disease, encephalographic and autonomic studies in dementia praecox, metabolism studies in psychoses, the use of color in the treatment of psychoses, and administrative technics as therapeutic agents in mental disorder. The productiveness of its staff members in original investigative work is reflected in its output of publications during the past three years: 33 in 1934, 29 in 1935, and 35 in 1936.

Worcester State Hospital would welcome additional funds to develop its research program on a broader front and in accordance with its long-range plans. At this time it is particularly interested in a further investigation of the rationale of insulin therapy, in studies of changes of electrical potential in the brain in schizophrenic and other mental conditions, and in investigations of early schizophrenia at its child guidance clinic. Approximately $50,000 a year, in addition to the funds at present available, could be expended advantageously for this purpose.

WRENTHAM STATE SCHOOL
Wrentham, Massachusetts

Wrentham State School is a relative newcomer in the field of psychiatric investigation, having set up a research department in 1936, in accordance with plans long in the making by its research-minded superintendent. It is one of the outstanding institutions in the country, with a fine record and tradition built up by the late Dr. George L. Wallace, who was for many years a nationally recognized leader in the field of mental deficiency. The Board, in its annual report, refers to the establishment of the Department of Research at this school as "the most forward step made in many years toward a better understanding of the many-sided problem of mental deficiency." And the superintendent writes, in the same report: "Research in the field of mental deficiency has been carried on to some extent in several institutions in this country and abroad, but no research unit has been established with personnel and equipment so complete as the one now being organized, capable of attacking the subject from pathological, bio-chemical and psychological, educational, social and other aspects.''

The research unit is housed in the new Children's Clinic Building which was built in 1932 for research purposes, and a state appropriation was recently made available for equipment and personnel. The pathological and bio-chemical equipment is complete, and research projects are already under way. The personnel thus far engaged includes a director of clinical psychiatry, who is in direct charge of all research activities; a bio-chemist; two laboratory technicians, and an x-ray technician. Although the director is a neuro-pathologist, it is planned to add a pathologist to the research staff when the volume of work becomes sufficient to warrant it. An addition to the clinical building, as it was originally planned, would provide for animal experimentation and for a small ward for a few children under study by the Research Department. This extension is not an immediate necessity but will be added within the next three years in order to complete the equipment for research work.

The institution has a patient population of about 2,000, with a yearly admission rate of about 200, and is clinically well organized and equipped for effective investigatory work. It has a medical staff of 11, a fairly large staff of nurses and attendants in proportion to the number of patients, a well-trained supervisor of occupational therapy, and two social workers. An out-patient clinic is held at the institution one day a week, with a psychiatrist, psychologist, school teacher and social worker available; and it also conducts a traveling (community) school clinic, with a psychiatrist and psychologist in charge.

There are no internes, but suitable arrangements are in effect for the training of the junior medical staff, with opportunities for experience in the reception and clinical services, out-patient clinics, laboratory and research department. A larger medical staff would increase the effectiveness of present training facilities. While there is no formal university affiliation, the superintendent lectures, from time to time, to classes from several Massachusetts colleges and universities. The institution has a fairly well stocked library, with 21 current journals, and, in addition, a special library is being formed in the research department.

Except for routine laboratory work, the staff of the department spends full time in research work. The department is fortunate in having the salaries of its personnel assured by state appropriation, so that in the future any gifts from private sources may be used for the purchase of materials for certain projects which would not be available through state appropriation. At least $5,000 a year, over and above its state budget, is needed to develop more complete studies than are now possible in the field of heredity, and for prolonged bio-chemical studies in the field of endocrinology.

Studies on heredity will be undertaken with the coöperation of the medical staff of the school and the social service department. A careful study will be made of the diseases of and accidents to the mother during the prenatal period, and of accidents and injuries occurring to the head during and after labor. Pathological studies will be made of tissues of the brain, ductless glands, and other organs in various types of mental deficiency, all of which should provide valuable information within the next ten years when the volume of material studied becomes sufficient to make reasonable deductions. Bio-chemical work will be undertaken particularly in reference to the relationship of the ductless gland system to mental deficiency; and a neurological study will be made of large numbers of children during their lifetime, which may be later correlated with post mortem findings. One paper on the pathological study of Mongoloids is ready for publication and others will follow as findings seem to warrant presentation.

The Neuropsychiatric Institute of the University Hospital

(Formerly State Psychopathic Hospital)

University of Michigan, Ann Arbor, Michigan

This institution was opened in 1906 and was the first university psychopathic hospital to be established in this country. It is essentially a teaching and research hospital, affiliated with the University of Michigan Medical School, and has long been a leading center of psychiatric education, with a broad and intensive training program. Regular instruction by both professional and nursing staff is given to undergraduate nurses of the University Hospital Training School. A center for graduate training in psychiatric nursing is planned. It conducts an out-patient department and has a staff of well-trained social service workers. Its laboratory facilities are good, with a pathologist, an assistant pathologist, and three technicians on duty. Examinations are made of nearly 1,000 neuropathologic specimens each year, a fairly large percentage of which come from the state hospitals of Michigan. It needs improved facilities for training purposes in neurophysiology and psychopathology, and also a special children's unit. It has an up-to-date library and commands reference facilities at the university library.

Eight of the ten members of its medical staff are actively engaged in research projects, of which the following are under way at the present time: clinical studies in schizophrenia, virus diseases, Lissauer's general paralysis, psychopathic personalities, puerperal psychosis, constitutional factors in psychoses, anthropometric measurements with objective evidence of body types, and electro-encephalography. A fund of $18,000 per year from the Rockefeller Foundation for laboratory training and work in a special unit in the university hospital ended July 1, 1937. This work is now being carried as a part of the hospital activity. Funds are desired for additional work along the following lines: producing experimental brain tumors, study of psychopathic personalities, correlation of body types, and electro-encephalography.

Several factors give promise of favorable developments in research work at this center within the next year or two, namely a high caliber of personnel, the significant character of the investigations now in progress, plans for new construction at the center and the contemplated establishment of a children's division to be closely linked with the university department of pediatrics, an increasing psychiatric-mindedness on the part of the other specialties in internal medicine, and a continuing tradition of high grade work in psychiatric teaching. A new unit of 83 beds, 20 of which are for children, is in process of construction and is expected to be completed by December 1, 1938. This will allow a much greater opportunity for both clinical and non-clinical research, for which funds are needed. Added to these developments are the plans for a comprehensive state hospital building program, the recent establishment of a promising state mental hygiene society, and other developments in enlarging the mental health resources of the State.

WAYNE COUNTY TRAINING SCHOOL
Northville, Michigan

This is one of the foremost schools for mental defectives in the country, with highly developed research interests. It has also an active training program and is in close touch with two university centers: University of Michigan and Wayne University. Regular instruction is given to undergraduate students in psychology, sociology, and education, and the opportunities for coöperative research work with these institutions are excellent. Students of speech psychology and sociology come to the school for special interneships and often use the material of the school for theses. One member of the school's staff, a psychologist, serves on the faculty of the University of Michigan.

The facilities of the school are well-rounded and equipped to serve its many-sided functions. The organization as a whole is divided into three main divisions: a mental-hygiene, health and cottage division; the school division; and the division of service and supply. Certain staff divisions, such as social service, concerning itself with both pre-admission investigation and after-care, vocational training supervision, and other community functions, work in liaison fashion. Ninety per cent of the patients receive occupational treatment and training.

Research is centralized in one division staffed by full- and part-time workers, two of whom have had special training in pediatrics and psychiatry. Its facilities are also used by other institutions, such as the University of Michigan Medical School and Graduate School of Social Work, and Harper Hospital. The physical plant, scientific outlook, resourcefulness and character of the personnel are excellent. And the attitude of the governmental authorities toward the institution's investigative activities is very coöperative.

Medical researches during the past three years dealt with such problems as nocturnal enuresis, increased sensitiveness in normal children produced by repeated injections of tuberculin, and active immunization with meningococcus toxin.

A long-term growth study has been under way for the past two years. The first year was devoted to repeated measurements with the establishment of curves for a given child and this year a very competent internist, with a thorough grounding in endocrine physiology, has been added to give the control to the treatment. Also in progress are a study of immunization against scarlet fever and another on immunization against gonococcus, an investigation of hyperinsulinism, and further tuberculin studies. The Research Department has also been strengthened by the recent addition of two independent workers: one in genetic psychology, the other in child psychopathology. One member of the medical staff is doing excellent work with reference to spontaneous drawings by children. Additional facilities are desired for anthropometric and biochemical research, and funds are needed for additional personnel, especially a full-time psychiatrist and a biochemist.

YPSILANTI STATE HOSPITAL
Ypsilanti, Michigan

This is the newest state hospital in Michigan, having been opened in 1931. It has a fair proportion of graduate nurses, an occupational therapy set-up serving about fifty per cent of the patients, good out-patient and social service arrangements, and good laboratory facilities. It is conveniently located for teaching purposes, being near the University of Michigan and the State Psychopathic Hospital at Ann Arbor. It trains one interne a year and, in addition, one to three third-year medical students receive training in summer months. It has a good library, well supplied with current texts and all the principal medical journals, and liberally supported from general appropriations.

Five of the physicians are interested in research, one of whom is a trained biochemist, and another well grounded in criminology. One devotes almost full time to research, and two others several hours a day. No special funds are available aside from those taken from the general budget. In this connection there is the encouraging observation that one newly appointed member of the State Hospital Commission is vitally interested in research work, and the belief that influence can be brought to bear upon the legislature in favor of public appropriations for research purposes. Worthy of note also is the outstanding quality of the medical staff and the progressive and alert character of its administration. Current research activities include a study of therapeutic effects of intensive clinical work with twenty-four dementia praecox cases using twenty-four controls; a study of blood sugar in manic states; metabolic studies in a case of encephalitis lethargica; encephalograms in dementia praecox cases; checking the results of treatment in syphilitic cases; outstanding tests applicable to psychotics; and an investigation of sera and anti-toxins. It would seem that Ypsilanti, because of good organization, scientific leadership, proximity to the University of Michigan, and other favorable factors, is a splendid center for psychiatric training and research.

Some $9,000 was spent on research projects during the past fiscal year, but considerably more is needed to develop the work. Probably $25,000 could profitably be used to expand the research staff and for further projects.

BELLEVUE PSYCHIATRIC HOSPITAL
New York, New York

This institution, which is a unit of Bellevue Hospital, operated by the City of New York, is the principal receiving center for mental cases in the metropolitan area and most of the patients admitted to the New York state hospitals from the area clear through this center. It is essentially an admission service for temporary care and observation. Unlike other psychopathic hospitals which provide continued treatment, it cannot, under the state law, keep its patients longer than thirty days. Actually the average length of stay is a little over eight days.

In spite of this limitation Bellevue Psychiatric Hospital has done notable therapeutic work and ranks high as a psychiatric clinic and research center. Its facilities are among the best in the country, thanks to the erection of its new building four years ago, though still somewhat short of their potential capacity and needs in service and equipment. It has an excellent staff of physicians, nurses, attendants, and occupational therapists, but these should be augmented by additional medical personnel and, especially, social service workers, to meet its optimum requirements.

The American Medical Association has recently approved the institution as a recognized training center in psychiatry, and with its exceptional resources, abundance of clinical material and competent leadership, the conditions are favorable to progressive achievement in scientific work, in training and research as well as in therapy.

In addition to the usual facilities of a psychopathic hospital it has a well-equipped medical and surgical service and enjoys the advantages that accrue to psychiatric departments of general hospitals in the command of special services in other branches of medicine. Other features are its special children's service, a prison ward, and an alcoholic ward. In addition to its in-patient services it conducts an out-patient mental hygiene clinic for adults and children, and a special clinic at the New York City Court of General Sessions. And there are well-equipped laboratories, with three full-time technicians, though laboratory work for the psychiatric department is done also in the division of pathology of the general hospital. Autopsies are performed in 30 per cent of the deaths among mental patients.

The various services are well utilized for professional training purposes, and twenty-five of the psychiatric staff members serve on the faculties of affiliated medical schools. There are twelve psychiatric internships and six residencies, all of which are one-year appointments. The internes spend their first six months on the quiet and semi-disturbed wards learning the general technique of examining patients. During their last six months their time is divided equally on the children's ward, the prison ward, and the disturbed wards. They also do work in the laboratories and it is planned to start special instruction in neuropathology for them in the near future. Students at the nursing school at Bellevue and Allied Hospitals all spend three months in training at the Psychiatric Hospital. A psychiatric library has just been installed.

Over half of the staff members engage in research work. Among the projects now in progress are those dealing with schizophrenia, with special reference to insulin and metrazol therapy; a study of the physiological changes occurring in blood chemistry during insulin coma; investigation of brain changes in alcoholism; experiments in vitamin therapy on alcoholics; studies in drug addiction, with special attention to psychoses due to bromides, barbiturates and alcohol; encephalographic studies; studies of brain injuries, brain trauma in the new-born, and the neurophysiology of vision.

New diagnostic and therapeutic measures have been adopted in the children's ward, which makes use of art and such novel devices as puppet shows and plastic molding. Other studies are concerned with form as a principle of play in children; play techniques in diagnosis and treatment; group music in the treatment of behavior disorders, dramatic work with adolescent girls, and other forms of group therapy; effects of intravenous injections of hypertonic saline solutions in stupors; grasping and kicking reflexes; and a personality analysis of criminal cases at the court clinic.

It is difficult to estimate the cost of most of these research activities as it is impossible to separate research from other work a great deal of the time. Among the projects separately financed is a special research on suicide, under a grant of $10,000 a year from the Committee for the Study of Suicide through New York University, which will be renewed for a second year. For the study of insulin and metrazol application is being made for a Foundation grant of $65,000 for a two-year research to further present investigations in this field. The Child Neurology Research Project of New York contributed to a study on brain metabolism in insulin cases, the results of which were recently published. And two research fellows are at work on special projects—one in the field of sex and the other on the mental changes produced by birth injuries. The hospital is also in quest of large funds for a long-term research in alcoholism, for which it is better equipped than perhaps any other hospital in the country.

LETCHWORTH VILLAGE
Thiells, New York

Letchworth Village is one of the few state schools for the feebleminded actively engaged in research work. It is one of the outstanding institutions, and one of the largest of its kind in this country, and represents the most modern conception of a program designed to secure better results in the socialization of the mentally deficient through segregation, classification, training, treatment and occupation, in a setting approximating as nearly as possible normal village life in a widely scattered community. Letchworth Village is at once a home, a laboratory and a school. It functions also as a hospital, with special departments as follows: out-patient, social service, dietetic, physical and occupational therapy, psychological, x-ray, clinical and pathological laboratories.

The nature of the institution and its nearness to educational and research centers in New York City afford unusual scientific and clinical opportunities. In addition to its regular training activities, it conducts, from time to time, a summer school to promote the study of mental deficiency by medical students and graduates, and to provide clinical and research training for qualified non-medical graduate students. It is approved for residency in its specialty by the American Medical Association, and would be able to train three or four internes a year. It draws upon the library facilities of the New York State Psychiatric Institute and the Academy of Medicine, and has some 800 volumes, including 20 periodicals, in its own library. On the other hand, it has no formal affiliation with a university center, and none of its staff serves on medical school faculties, though it hopes to develop such contacts in the future.

Three of the staff members devote practically all of their time to research. They are quartered in a separate research building and have excellent laboratory facilities at their disposal. Three technicians are employed, and an autopsy rate of 40 per cent is a significant index of the institution's pathological activities. Some thirty original papers have been published or accepted for publication from seven staff members during the past three years. Considerable attention is given to the problem of securing well trained people capable of assisting in the development of sound clinical work, which is the basis for sound educational and research activities in the institution. The research members in joint consultation diagnose all new admissions, the diagnoses being classified under medical, neurological, psychological and psychiatric headings.

The research department consists of four divisions: psychiatry, neurology and neuropathology, psychology, and auxology; and it has the benefit of advisory services from a Research Council composed of leading specialists outside the institution. We quote the following statement of policy of the department from the institution's annual report for 1936: "The past year has witnessed the appearance of an enlarged concept of the field in which we are working and the production of work which has contributed toward the reality-testing of theoretical considerations in our research. In brief, the field of mental deficiency has been viewed essentially as the field of developmental deficiency, since variously determined deficiencies in the growth and development of the organism may be found in different combinations in the physical, intellectual, emotional and social aspects of the organism. As a medical field, the field of developmental deficiency requires, in addition to the work of the physician, the closest coöperation with the geneticist, the auxologist, the neurologist, psychologist, psychiatrist, sociologist and educator. Not only is there the need for the development of more effective custodianship but also for therapy, and especially for research and prevention. The goal-idea before our department is the finding of processes through which the problems of deficiency may be controlled and reduced in their personal, social and economic aspects, and through the approach to such a goal, the attainment of methods and other procedures which may be utilized in establishing an optimum life-milieu for average and superior children.''

During the past year work has gone forward on the study of personality, character and behavior of developmentally deficient children, and further progress in this field waits upon the development of a more complete psychiatric service, which it is hoped will be available in the near future. In the division of neurology and neuropathology extensive research activities have been carried on in the following fields: encephalographic studies of the mentally or developmentally deficient; studies of the nature of tuberous sclerosis; phenylpuruvic oligophrenia or Fölling's Disease; and the cytoarchitectonics of mental deficiency. The latter is new work in a virgin field. In connection with the research on oligophrenia, the investigator reports the interesting finding that this type appears to act as a Mendelian recessive sparing entirely Jews and Negroes. Other researches of this division have been carried on in collaboration with the Psychiatric Institute and Hospital. Work in auxology is in progress in coöperation with the Carnegie Institution for Genetics, with special reference to physical anthropometry. This work is of growing importance as a significant basis for the investigation of certain fundamental aspects of the growth and development of children.

The division of psychology has been making a comparative study of various intelligence tests, in an attempt to arrive at a better understanding of the ultimate meaning of these tests, and to provide for more effective examination. Research studies include also investigation of occupational aptitudes at various mental-age levels, and studies using an observation-room technique. The records of routine and special examinations are all being kept in such form that they can readily be used for research purposes.

About $30,000, or 2.7 per cent of the institution's total budget, is charged up to the research department. Of this amount, an estimated $12,000, or 1.1 per cent of the total budget, goes into actual research work.

NEW YORK STATE PSYCHIATRIC INSTITUTE AND HOSPITAL
Columbia Medical Center, New York City

The establishment of the Psychiatric Institute is the outcome of a fortunate combination of circumstances whereby an opportunity was afforded in 1923 for coöperation between the State of New York and the Medical Department of Columbia University which was then building its great medical center. The necessary legislation was enacted and as a result the New York State Psychiatric Institute and Hospital is most favorably placed as an affiliated unit in the largest and probably the most active medical center in the world. The Institute preserves its identity as a unit built and financed by the State of New York and in its teaching and scientific work has intimate association with the other units and departments of the medical center. This affords a splendid chance for the personal contact of its staff with clinicians and research workers in practically all other branches of medicine, many of which overlap the field of psychiatry and present many problems of mutual interest.

The Psychiatric Institute is the scientific nerve center of the New York state hospital system and has exerted a marked influence on the development of scientific work in all of the State's mental hospitals. It has an operating budget of about $500,000 per annum and is adequately equipped and staffed for diagnostic, therapeutic, teaching and research purposes. It has a splendid medical library: some 5,000 books and 7,000 volumes of journals, including

300 different periodicals in various languages. About $5,000 a year is spent on books, journals and other library activities.

The building of the Institute is a twenty-story structure. There are two hundred and ten beds for patients and living accommodations are provided for a hundred workers. In general the wards and personnel quarters are all below the tenth floor: the out-patient clinic, administrative offices, library, museum, and laboratories are on the ten upper floors.

For purposes of description, the internal organization of the Institute may be visualized as having four divisions, namely, (1) a hospital and out-patient division; (2) a clinical research division; (3) a laboratory research division, and (4) an accounting and maintenance division. The hospital and out-patient division comprises male and female hospital departments, an out-patient department, a department of nursing, a social service department, a department of occupational therapy and a department of physiotherapy, all with special provisions for children.

With the hospital and out-patient division supplying the problems for psychiatric research, the clinical research division and the laboratory research division are furnished with a constant source of material. The latitude which has been given the director in the selection of clinical cases makes it possible to concentrate at any one time all the resources on the investigation of some major research problem. The facilities for research are therefore exceptional.

The clinical research division consists of a department of clinical psychiatry headed by a research associate in psychiatry, a department of clinical medicine headed by a research associate in internal medicine, and a department of clinical and laboratory psychology, headed by a research associate in psychology.

The laboratory research division consists of three departments: neuroanatomy and neuropathology, chem-

istry, and bacteriology, each directed by a research associate. None of these research laboratory departments is
handicapped by routine laboratory demands of the hospital or out-patient division. In addition to these six
research associates, the staff includes three research
assistants.

The nucleus of the medical staff of the hospital and out-
patient department consists of the director and assistant
director, a research associate in psychiatry, five full-time
psychiatrists and five internes, with additional consulting
specialists and physicians taking post-graduate work.

In developing its research program the Institute has
followed a coördinated scheme and plan in which the
diverse activities of its various departments fit together
and which, it is felt, will shed progressively new light on
the varied and sundry abnormalities of the psychobiology
of the individual. While the Institute functions as the
research center of the New York state hospitals, the
director does not regard it as the exclusive place for such
activity but seeks to stimulate research work in all of the
state hospitals, and to integrate the separate researches
in the individual institutions with the Institute's own
program.

This program is very full at the present time, with 38
distinct projects under way. Of these, 17 are along basic
scientific lines and may apply in several directions in
medicine. Psychiatry is thus identified with the medical
sciences and the value of fundamental scientific work is
recognized, whether or not it has any immediate bearing
on the specific problem under consideration. There are,
however, so many matters of immediate and practical
interest in dealing with patients and so many obscurities
in the etiology of their conditions that more than 20
research studies have to do with living patients and their
problems and situations.

In the department of internal medicine one of the major
activities is concerned with the hormone question and

this department has entered several of the fields which have to do with the internal secretions. Another major problem constitutes the study of insulin therapy in cases of dementia praecox. Other studies are being carried on in connection with polycythemia associated with encephalitis manifestations; the administration of hematoporphyrin in cases of depression; and the therapeutic and metabolic effects of vitamin therapy in a severe case of pellagra.

In the department of bacteriology the major problem has been concerned with general and cerebral anaphylaxis in the monkey, with special interest in the quantitative aspects in cerebral anaphylaxis. The importance of the morphological type upon the physiological function of bacteria is being investigated. In the immediate future the influence of hormones and vitamins on antibody production and anaphylaxis, with particular reference to the possible role of anaphylaxis in epilepsy, will be studied.

In the department of clinical psychiatry general paresis is being studied with special attention to serological changes and reactions to therapeutic procedures; the psychology of the manic phase of the manic-depressive psychoses was investigated and recently published; a study of the manic-depressive reaction in adolescence is contemplated; and an investigation is being made into the parotid secretory rate in psychiatric patients.

In the children's hospital service a study is being made of the present status of all children formerly hospitalized; various new technical approaches that could be used in the study and treatment of emotional problems in children are now being investigated; and special problems in schizophrenia and in epilepsy are under investigation.

In the department of psychology psychosexual development, personality traits and configurations have constituted an outstanding group problem; an investigation is under way concerning the social significance of mental disease; the pattern of response which takes place as the immediate reflex following the sound of a pistol shot is being studied with high speed motion picture photography; an investigation of concept formation in psychopathic individuals has been undertaken; and in addition to these problems the department has sponsored graduate work in abnormal psychology in Columbia University.

In the department of chemistry the studies on the gonadal-stimulating hormones have been undertaken in coöperation with the departments of internal medicine and clinical psychiatry. Other investigations consist of metabolic and therapeutic studies in the myopathies; brain metabolism; intermediary protein and sulfur metabolism; and brain proteins.

In the department of neuropathology the following conditions are being studied: arsphenamine encephalopathy; Pick's disease; alcoholism and vitamin deficiency; demyelinizing processes of the central nervous system; experimental phosphorus poisoning; brain wound; arteriosclerosis; experimental phenol poisoning; the anatomy and effects of lesions of the nucleus lateralis of the medulla; electrical and anatomical phenomena associated with the response of the cochlea of the cat to sound; and experimental neurology with emphasis on studies of the sensory system.

Also under way is a study on the specific construction of tissues with their reactions to various diseases in the two main groups of mental disorders; and the effect on the embryo of various growth-promoting or growth-inhibiting substances is being studied.

By attacking the complex and interrelated problems of mental disorder, constitutional and metabolic pathology directly and indirectly · in these various types of approaches, it is hoped that important contributions to psychiatry will be made and also new scientific techniques devised that may be used to advantage in the medical sciences in general.

COLUMBUS STATE HOSPITAL
Columbus, Ohio

This is one of the more progressive state hospitals of Ohio and promises to develop into a significant research and training center. Plans are now shaping for an interne training program on a rotating service basis, and several residencies in psychiatry have been established. The residents in psychiatry are graduates who have completed their interneship and who are there to spend another year in training. In addition, there are three externes, senior medical students who spend full time at the hospital during the summer, and evenings and week-ends during the school year.

The department of pathology is actively associated with the Ohio State University. The establishment of a department of neuropsychology at the hospital is contemplated. Plans are also in prospect for an enlarged out-patient and social service department, more occupational therapy, and a program of psychiatric training for nurses. The laboratory arrangements are good, and there is a library of 1,400 books and 18 periodicals.

Four members of the staff show keen research inclinations, but routine duties limit the time they can devote to research activity under present conditions. The superintendent, recently appointed, reports that his "main interest is research," and hopes "very much to stimulate the research activities in this hospital." He further states: "I expect all my staff members to be interested in research in some form, and promotions will be made in accordance with their interest in active psychiatric research." Present staff interests run to the following: blood sedimentation in dementia praecox; endocrinology (physique and personality); differential diagnoses of schizophrenia and schizophrenic types; cerebral frontal agenesis not associated with epilepsy; fever therapy; sodium amytal narcosis; alcoholism; and organic psychiatry.

The hospital anticipates having twelve students from the various departments of Ohio State University doing active research during the coming months. A number of them will be working in the hospital toward their Ph.D. at the university. Two students from the Department of Genetics have begun special work at the hospital, also some advanced students from the Medical Department who are interested in some long-time research work. According to indications, the possibilities for research activity at the hospital look very promising for the near future.

Very little has actually been spent thus far for research work, though various purchases of equipment have been made to lay the ground-work for research purposes, and additional funds will be required.

WISCONSIN PSYCHIATRIC INSTITUTE
Madison, Wisconsin

This institution serves as the Department of Neuropsychiatry of the state-owned Wisconsin General Hospital and is the principal center for psychiatric research in the state. It is located in the University of Wisconsin Medical School, the director serving as chairman of the department of neuropsychiatry, and six other staff members as professors, assistant professors and instructors of neuropsychiatry. It trains twelve internes a year, on a rotating service. An active connection is also maintained with the State Hospital of Mendota, near Madison, where the fourth-year medical students obtain their ward training in psychiatry. Psychiatric instruction is also given at the university school of nursing. In addition, one of the instructors from the department devotes half time to the university student mental health service.

While the Department of Neuropsychiatry is an integral part of the Wisconsin General Hospital, it is housed in a separate building, but using all the laboratory and special facilities of the main building. Its present physical set-up is far from adequate, and the building used is a temporary arrangement until such time as the legislature appropriates funds for proper equipment. This is expected to be the first expansion in the medical school. The laboratory service of the Psychiatric Institute is housed in the same building which houses the department, the funds for the operation of which come from the State General Fund. (The salaries of part of the staff of the department are paid from the Psychiatric Institute budget, the others by the medical school.) The funds for the Institute are appropriated by the University of Wisconsin whose budget comes directly from the legislature.

A most important function of the Psychiatric Institute is its free laboratory service for the physicians of Wisconsin. Blood Wassermanns, complete spinal fluid examinations, and blood chemistry studies are made upon specimens sent in by physicians from all parts of the state. The laboratory facilities for the department of neuropsychiatry are excellent and are part of the laboratory system of the Wisconsin General Hospital. Post-mortems are done on 70 to 80 per cent of the deaths in the Wisconsin General Hospital, which includes those in the Department of Neuropsychiatry. This is part of the service of the pathology department of the medical school, presided over by the professor of pathology.

The Department of Neuropsychiatry has an average of 50 resident patients, with a turn-over of about 1,000 cases a year. Approximately 40 per cent of these are purely psychiatric, the remainder neurological. It is mainly a diagnostic service, although the average hospital residence of 18 days indicates that a number of patients are held for treatment. An active consultation system is maintained by the various departments of the Wisconsin General Hospital, and patients are freely transferred from one department to another.

The Institute maintains an active out-patient service. While it has no social worker of its own, it secures satisfactory case studies from the various social and governmental agencies, from which most of the out-patient cases are referred.

The Institute at one time had its own library, but in recent years only a limited number of periodicals have been subscribed to, since there are available to the Institute the resources of an excellent medical school library.

Five members of the Institute's medical staff are actively interested in research, and devote a third of their time to research work. Active work has been done during the past three years on tryparsamide, malaria and artificial fever treatment, encephalography, sodium amytal narcosis, and other drug therapies. Funds for investigative work are limited, the absence of adequate financial resources prohibiting the employment of the desired number of qualified investigators, in spite of the liberal aids to laboratory work available at the university, and other advantages. The state hospital at Mendota, for example, provides ample clinical material.

Work is now in progress on insulin treatment in schizophrenia, and two of the staff are working on the antidotal action of picrotoxin in barbiturate intoxication. Funds are required for further studies of insulin therapy and for the improvement of serological procedures; and special interest is manifested in an investigation of the relation of climate to mental disease.

PART IV

EVALUATION OF BASIC FACILITIES IN TAX-SUPPORTED INSTITUTIONS

CONTENTS

Part IV

Evaluation of Basic Facilities in State Hospitals and Other Tax-Supported Institutions

INTRODUCTION: SCOPE, METHOD AND RESULTS OF APPRAISAL

T HE questionnaire on research facilities consisted of 24 items. These included many questions about the hospital facilities that did not deal with research as such but which had considerable bearing, directly or indirectly, on the type and caliber of the research conducted in certain institutions and on the opportunities for research presented by certain other institutions. The responses to these questions were tabulated item by item. These items are presented in the accompanying tables and their distribution for the state hospitals and other types of hospitals is given.

The vast proportions of the problem of mental disease can be realized by inspecting Tables I and II. There are about half a million patients in institutions of all types for mental disease and for mental defect and epilepsy. Of this number, 97.1 per cent are in government-controlled institutions and only 2.9 per cent in privately controlled institutions. These patients are hospitalized in 603 institutions of which 247 or 41 per cent are under private control and 366 or 59.7 per cent are under governmental control.

The present survey dealt only with the government-controlled institutions for mental disease and mental defect and epilepsy, of which there are 356.* After some preliminary investigation, 83 institutions were eliminated because of their apparent lack of research facilities. Questionnaires were sent to the remaining 273.

Of the 273 institutions to which questionnaires were sent, 224 returned questionnaires. Six of the institutions that

---

* Since the study was limited to institutions for mental disease, mental defect and epilepsy, institutions for drug addicts such as the United States Narcotic Farm at Lexington, Kentucky, although they are engaged in important research, were not included.

TABLE I

DISTRIBUTION OF PATIENTS IN AVERAGE DAILY RESIDENCE IN INSTITUTIONS OF THE UNITED STATES, BY TYPE OF INSTITUTION

Type of Institution	Hospitals for Mental Disease	Psychopathic Hospitals	Institutions for Mental Defectives and Epileptics	Institutions for Alcoholics and Drug Addicts	Total
UNDER GOVERMENT CONTROL...	406,646	485	93,962	758	501,851
State.	348,366(a)	449	92,058(c)	...	440,873
County.	27,180(b)	...	662	...	27,842
City.	4,709	36	1,242(d)	...	5,987
Veterans Administration Facilities and Federal......	26,391	...	......	758	27,149
UNDER PRIVATE CONTROL.....	11,948	335	3,220	48	15,551
Non-Profit.	6,529(e)#	223	2,519	15	9,286
Proprietary.	5,419(f)#	112	701(g)	33	6,265
GRAND TOTAL	418,594	820	97,182	806	517,402

Source: Hospital Number of the Journal of the American Medical Association, March, 1937 (also March 1936).
  # Patients with mental disease in private hospitals are classified under three headings: nervous and mental, mental, or nervous. The total of these three classifications has been given.
  No figures were available for 1936 for 39 institutions. For 31 of these, the 1935 figures were used. For the remaining 8, the number of beds was used.
  (a) Includes 1935 figures for 2 institutions and number of beds for one institution.
  (b) Includes 1935 figures for 7 institutions.
  (c) Includes 1935 figures for 3 institutions.
  (d) Includes 1935 figures for 1 institution.
  (e) Includes 1935 figures for 3 institutions.
  (f) Includes 1935 figures for 12 institutions and number of beds for 7 institutions.
  (g) Includes 1935 figures for 3 institutions.

TABLE II

MENTAL INSTITUTIONS IN THE UNITED STATES, BY TYPE OF INSTITUTION, 1936

Type of Institution	Hospitals for Mental Disease	Psychopathic Hospitals	Institutions for Mental Defectives and Epileptics	Institutions for Alcoholics and Drug Addicts	Total
UNDER GOVERNMENT CONTROL.....	266	7	82	1	356
State. .'	172	6	78	..	256
County.	62	..	1	..	63
City.	5	1	3	..	9
Veterans Administration Facilities and Federal.	27	..	..	1	28
UNDER PRIVATE CONTROL.........	213	2	25	7	247
Non-Profit.	39	1	10	1	51
Proprietary.	174	1	15	6	196
GRAND TOTAL.	479	9	107	8	603

Source: Hospital Number of the Journal of the American Medical Association, March 1937 (also March 1936).

made returns were placed in a miscellaneous group, and four more returned questionnaires with insufficient information. The questionnaires of the remaining 214 were analyzed. The distribution of these 214 institutions by type and by region is shown in Table III.

TABLE III

INSTITUTIONS PARTICIPATING IN SURVEY, BY TYPE AND REGION *

Type	New England	Middle Atlantic	East North Central	West North Central	South Atlantic	East South Central	West South Central	Mountain	Pacific	Total
State Hospital	13	28	29	17	14	5	8	6	7	127
Psychiatric and Psychopathic Hospitals	1	3	4	1	0	0	1	1	0	11
Institutions for Mental Defectives and Epileptics	8	14	9	9	5	1	2	3	2	53
Veterans Administration Facilities	2	4	5	1	3	2	2	2	2	23
Total	24	49	47	28	22	8	13	12	11	214

* For the individual States in each region see Appendix B.

Two of the institutions included in this survey were county hospitals and they have been classified with the state hospitals for mental disease. There were 127 state hospitals, 11 psychiatric and psychopathic hospitals, 23 Veterans Administration Facilities and Federal hospitals, and 53 state institutions for mental defectives and epileptics.

In an attempt to arrive at a single index of the relative status of each institution with regard to research facilities, each of the questionnaire items was evaluated on a scale, and the total scale score for each institution was obtained. The scale values were determined, perforce, arbitrarily on *a priori* grounds. Thus, for the item dealing with medical personnel, the ratio of patients to physicians in the hospital was taken as an index of the adequacy of medical personnel. Since the American Psychiatric Association has established a ratio of 150 patients to each physician as a maximum patient load, hospitals that live up to this standard received the maximum weighted rating for this item—9. Hospitals that had a patient load between 151 and 220 received a rating of 8 and so on.

Each item was evaluated in a similar way. In order to validate the scale values given to each item, 32 hospitals that were considered definitely unsuited for research were compared on each item with 32 hospitals in which research facilities were quite good. If the item in question proved its worth by giving a better average rating to the "good" than to the "poor" institutions, it was retained. If, on the other hand, the "poor" institutions achieved a higher or equal rating to that of the "good" institutions, the item was eliminated. This analysis was carried out for the state hospitals only, since some standards are available for evaluating the administration of these hospitals, and no standards have ever been established for the other types of institutions.

The general findings of the study indicate first, that the plan for rating hospitals utilized in this study proved to be a suitable method for evaluating hospitals in general and research possibilities in particular. The ratings obtained for the individual hospitals show a marked correlation with the impressions and evaluations of the surveyors.

Second, good hospitals and good research facilities are more frequently found in certain regions of the country than in others. The better types of hospitals are more frequently found in the New England and Middle Atlantic States; the poorer types of hospitals in the Mountain and East South Central States.

I. RATINGS OF THE STATE HOSPITALS

Table IV shows the distribution of total weighted ratings for all the state hospitals that were surveyed. The total range of weighted ratings was from 5 through 55

TABLE IV

Distribution of the Research Ratings for State Hospitals, by Regions

Crude Ratings (66 maximum)	New England	Middle Atlantic	East North Central	West North Central	South Atlantic	East South Central	West South Central	Mountain	Pacific	Total	Per Cent	Standard Ratings (100 maximum)
51–55		1								1	0.8	76.5–82.5
46–50	1	3	2				1			7	5.5	69.0–75.0
41–45	4	12	4		1	2	2			25	19.7	61.5–67.5
36–40	1	9	4	3	1					18	14.2	54.0–60.0
31–35	2	2	7	5	3	2	1	1	1	24	18.9	46.5–52.5
26–30	1	1	5	4	1			1	2	15	11.8	39.0–45.0
21–25	3		3	2	2	1	1	1	2	15	11.8	31.5–37.5
16–20	1		2	2	3		3	1	1	13	10.2	24.0–30.0
11–15			2	1	3			1	1	8	6.3	16.5–22.5
6–10								1		1	0.8	9.0–15.0
Total	13	28	29	17	14	5	8	6	7	127	100.	

with one hospital at each end. The ratings for the remaining hospitals distributed themselves rather unevenly between these two extremes, with a slight excess of the higher ratings than of the lower ratings. The predominance of the higher ratings is probably due to the selection of the better hospitals for the survey, since about 40 of the poorer hospitals were eliminated at the outset. In order to simplify the scale, the maximum rating, which was 66, was stepped up to 100, and the remaining ratings were expressed as percentages of 66. The crude rating based on a maximum of 66 is given in the left hand margin of Table IV and the stepped-up rating, or standard rating, is given in the right hand margin.

TABLE V

RANK ORDER OF REGIONS BY RATINGS

	Crude Median (Based on maximum of 66 points)	Standard Median (Based on 100 points)
Middle Atlantic.	41.8	63.3
New England.	34.8	52.7
East North Central	32.7	49.5
West North Central	30.4	46.1
Pacific.	29.8	45.2
West South Central	26.0	39.4
South Atlantic.	23.5	35.6
Mountain.	21.0	31.8
East South Central	19.8	30.0
United States.	33.8	51.2

Table V shows the regions in the order of median ratings. It will be noted that the Middle Atlantic and the New England States are close to the top while the East South Central and the Mountain States are at the lower end.

II. ANALYSIS OF INDIVIDUAL QUESTIONNAIRE ITEMS

The items of the questionnaire have been subdivided into the following five groups: Capacity and Occupancy of Institutions; Personnel; Clinical Facilities; Teaching

Facilities; and Research Facilities. Each of these groups will be treated separately in the following pages. Wherever the questionnaire failed to give some pertinent data for computing a given index of hospital care, the median index for the region in which the hospital was located, was utilized. This was done in order to render all the hospital ratings comparable.

The general findings in the five areas of hospital facilities can be summarized as follows:

A. Capacity and Occupancy of Institutions

The data available for the capacity of institutions did not prove to be comparable in the various states and the measures of occupancy and overcrowding were, therefore, not utilized in the ratings.

B. Adequacy of Personnel

The adequacy of the personnel varied considerably from region to region and from one type of hospital to another. Generally, the Veterans Administration Facilities were the most adequately equipped from the point of view of personnel. Next in order were the state hospitals and last—the institutions for mental defectives and epileptics. There was considerable variation between the regions in the adequacy of personnel in state hospitals, the best equipped regions being the New England and Middle Atlantic, while the least equipped were the South Central and Mountain Regions.

Occupational therapy and social work are not as highly developed in some regions as in others. Only 76 per cent of the state hospitals had occupational therapists and only 65 per cent reported having social workers.

The psychopathic and psychiatric hospitals are not compared with the others, since they are quite different in general purpose from the other institutions.

C. Clinical Facilities

With regard to clinical facilities, the Veterans Administration Facilities and the psychiatric and psychopathic hospitals were found to head the list and the institutions for mental defectives were at the bottom.

The superiority of the Middle Atlantic and New England Regions with regard to clinical facilities was not as marked as in the other items. The Pacific, the East North Central and West North Central States excelled the eastern regions in some of the items covered under the category of clinical facilities.

D. Teaching Facilities

The institutions that have the most adequate teaching facilities are, of course, the psychopathic and psychiatric hospitals. All these institutions have university contacts while 58 per cent of the state hospitals for mental disease, 53 per cent of the state institutions for mental defectives and only 35 per cent of the Veterans Administration Facilities have university contacts.

More than one-half of the state hospitals have no internes and more than one-third have no junior medical staff. In only one-fourth is a rotating service instituted.

E. Research Facilities

The staffs of the psychiatric and psychopathic hospitals are reported to have the largest proportions of research-interested men. The Veterans Administration Facilities report the lowest proportion of research-interested men. The proportion of research-interested men in the state hospitals for mental disease and the state institutions for mental defectives and epileptics is about the same—20 per cent.

The region that has the highest proportion of

research-interested men is the West North Central, the region with the lowest proportion is the Mountain Region.

A little less than half of all the institutions reported research interests in the psychiatric and neurological field. About one-eighth reported research interests in the field of general medicine. About one-third of all the institutions reported no research interests whatsoever.

About one-fourth of the state hospitals reported that they had no physical facilities for research.

A. CAPACITY AND OCCUPANCY OF INSTITUTIONS

The capacity and percentage occupancy of an institution are important considerations in its research program. Institutions that are very small do not have a sufficiently diverse number of patients to permit extensive research. The degree of occupancy is important, for, in institutions that are overcrowded, research can not be carried on smoothly or efficiently. Furthermore, the basic needs of the patient must be met before scientific research can be introduced. At the present time, adequate figures on overcrowding are not available in many institutions. Although most of the institutions report their bed capacities, the latter are usually based not on standard space requirements per patient, but either on the number of beds that can be crowded into the wards, or, sometimes, simply on the number of patients actually in the hospital during the previous year. For this reason, the data on overcrowding were not utilized in the total rating of the hospital.

More complete figures than those afforded by the present survey for overcrowding are given by the data of the Bureau of the Census. These figures, too, suffer from a lack of accuracy and uniformity in the estimate of rated capacity. The data for geographic regions are shown in Table VI.

TABLE VI

AVERAGE DAILY RESIDENT PATIENT POPULATION AND NORMAL CAPACITY
OF STATE HOSPITALS, 1935

	Average Daily Resident Patient Population	Normal Capacity	Excess of Population Over Capacity	
			Number	Per cent
New England.	32,740	28,314	4,426	15.6
Middle Atlantic.	86,136	77,102	9,034	11.7
East North Central.	67,603	63,637	3,966	6.2
West North Central.	34,830	30,850	3,980	12.9
South Atlantic.	42,209	28,858	3,351	8.6
East South Central.	19,162	17,295	1,867	10.8
West South Central.	26,853	24,164	2,689	11.1
Mountain.	9,448	8,773	675	7.7
Pacific.	28,639	23,165	5,474	23.6
United States.	347,620	312,158	35,462	11.4

Source: "Patients in Hospitals for Mental Disease," Bureau of the Census. United States Department of Commerce, U. S. Government Printing Office, Wash., D. C., 1935.

The region with the highest degree of reported over-crowding is the Pacific Region with 23.6 per cent over-crowding above capacity, while the lowest degree of overcrowding is found in the East North Central region.

B. PERSONNEL

The personnel of the institutions consists of the medical staff, nursing staff, occupational therapists, social workers and others. The adequacy of the staff is determined by calculating the patient load on each staff member. In the case of occupational therapists and social workers, since the entire patient population is not served by them, the patient load is not a suitable index, but it has been retained as an index of adequacy in the absence of any better measure.

1. Medical Staff

The best available index of the adequacy of medical personnel is the patient load per assistant physician.* Table

* The ratio of patients to medical personnel does not include the superintendent because he is regarded as devoting most of his time to administrative duties and not to therapy.

VII shows the distribution of the ratio of patients to assistant physicians in the hospitals that were surveyed. The
median state hospital had a patient load of 293.4 patients
per assistant physician. There were 9 hospitals that had
a load in excess of 500 patients per assistant physician
while 7 hospitals had less than 150 patients per assistant
physician.

The ratio of patients to assistant physicians in the
median hospital of the Veterans Administration Facilities was 89.3. There the range was from 50 to 140
patients per assistant physician. There were three hospitals with less than 60 patients per assistant physician
and three hospitals with more than 120 patients per
assistant physician. For one hospital data were not
available.

The psychopathic hospitals, of course, have the lowest
ratio of patients to assistant physician. There the ratio

TABLE VII

PATIENT LOAD PER ASSISTANT PHYSICIAN IN MENTAL INSTITUTIONS

Patient Load	State Hospitals		Psychopathic and Psychiatric Hospitals		Institutions for Mental Defectives and Epileptics		Veterans Administration Facilities		Weighted Ratings
	No.	%	No.	%	No.	%	No.	%	
711.	5	3.9			5	9.4			0
641–710.	1	0.8			1	1.9			1
571–640.	1	0.8			6	11.3			2
501–570.	2	1.6			8	15.1			3
431–500.	9	7.1			8	15.1			4
361–430.	17	13.4			8	15.1			5
291–360.	29	22.8			4	7.5			6
221–290.	22	17.3			4	7.5			7
151–220.	33	26.0			3	5.7			8
101–150.	7	5.5			1	1.9	8	34.8	9
50–100.	0	0.0	9	81.8	1	1.9	14	60.8	9
Less than 50.	0	0.0			0	0.0	0	0.0	9
Not stated.	1	0.8	2	18.2	4	7.5	1	4.4	*
Total.	127	100.	11	100.	53	100.	23	100.	
Median.	293.4		9		461.6		89.3		

* Regional Median.

GRAPH 2

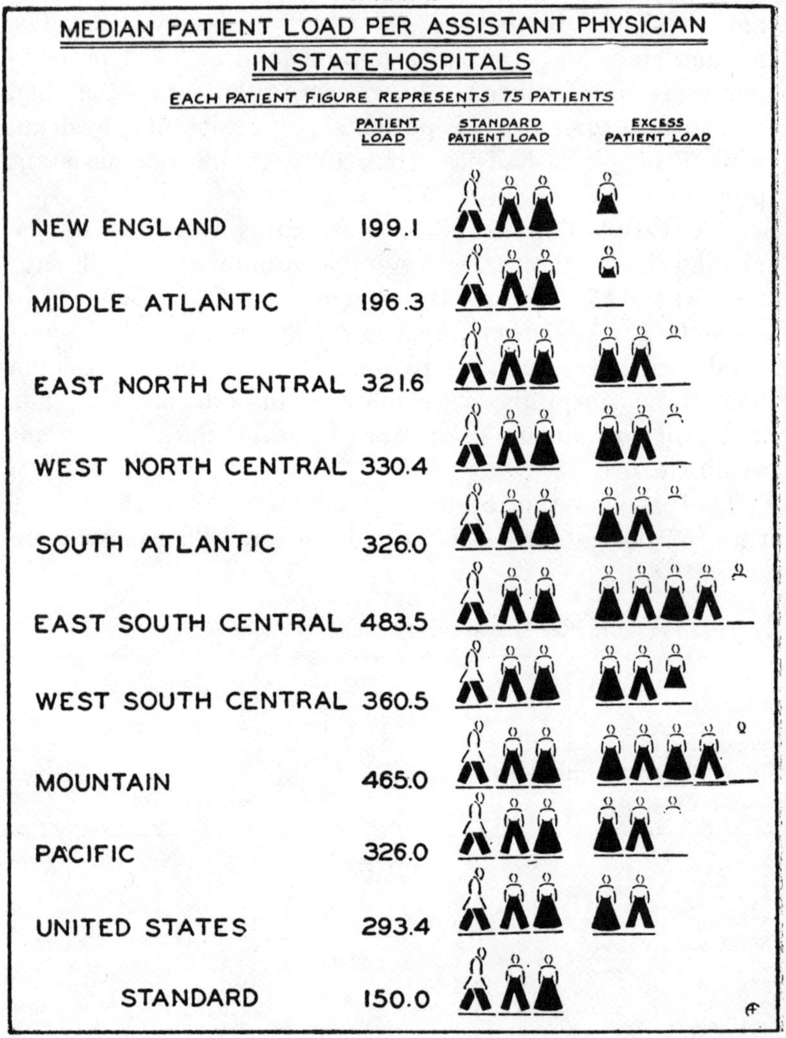

MEDIAN PATIENT LOAD PER ASSISTANT PHYSICIAN
IN STATE HOSPITALS

EACH PATIENT FIGURE REPRESENTS 75 PATIENTS

	PATIENT LOAD	STANDARD PATIENT LOAD	EXCESS PATIENT LOAD
NEW ENGLAND	199.1		
MIDDLE ATLANTIC	196.3		
EAST NORTH CENTRAL	321.6		
WEST NORTH CENTRAL	330.4		
SOUTH ATLANTIC	326.0		
EAST SOUTH CENTRAL	483.5		
WEST SOUTH CENTRAL	360.5		
MOUNTAIN	465.0		
PACIFIC	326.0		
UNITED STATES	293.4		
STANDARD	150.0		

ranges from 10 to 40, with two hospitals having a ratio of 30 or more patients per assistant physician and five hospitals having a ratio as low as 10. The median hospital has a ratio of 9 patients per assistant physician.

In the institutions for mental defectives and epileptics,

the ratio of patients to assistant physician ranged from 100 to more than 1,000. There were 13 institutions with a ratio of 300 or less patients per assistant physician while about 12 hospitals had a ratio of 600 or more patients per assistant physician. The ratio in the median hospital was 461.6 patients per assistant physician.

TABLE VIII

MEDIAN PATIENT LOAD PER ASSISTANT PHYSICIAN
IN STATE HOSPITALS, BY REGIONS

	Number of Hospitals	Number of Patients per Assistant Physician
New England.	13	199.1
Middle Atlantic.	28	196.3
East North Central.	29	321.6
West North Central.	17	330.4
South Atlantic.	14	326.0
East South Central.	5	483.5
West South Central.	8	360.5
Mountain.	6	465.0
Pacific.	7	326.0
Total.	127	293.4

The ratio of patients to assistant physicians in state hospitals by regional areas is shown in Table VIII. The regions in which the median hospital had the lowest patient load per assistant physician were New England and the Middle Atlantic Region. The regions with the heaviest load were the Mountain and East South Central States.

2. Nursing Staff

According to the standards of the American Psychiatric Association, the patient load per nurse and attendant should not exceed eight. The patient load by regional areas is shown in Table IX. The median state hospital does not live up to the standards of the American Psychiatric Association. The patient load in the median hospital is 11.8, or 47.5 per cent in excess of the standard load. Only 32 hospitals, or 25 per cent of the total, live

TABLE IX

PATIENT LOAD PER NURSE AND ATTENDANT IN THE STATE HOSPITALS FOR MENTAL DISEASE, BY REGIONS

Patient Load	New England	Middle Atlantic	East North Central	West North Central	South Atlantic	East South Central	West South Central	Mountain	Pacific	Total	Per cent	Weighted Ratings
25–28		1						1	1	3	2.4	4
21–24					2		2		1	5	3.9	5
17–20	1	1	2	4	2	3	1	2		16	12.6	6
13–16	1	1	8	5	6	2			3	26	20.5	7
9–12	4	10	13	5	3		5	2	2	44	34.6	8
8 and under	7	15	6	2	1			1		32	25.2	9
Not stated				1**						1	0.8	*
Total	13	28	29	17	14	5	8	6	7	127	100.	
Regional Median	8.0	8.0	11.4	13.8	15.0	17.7	12.2	15.0	15.0	11.8		

* Regional Median.

** Anoka State Asylum, Minnesota—Nursing Personnel unknown.

Source: Figures for New York State Hospitals were obtained from Annual Report of Department of Mental Hygiene, 1936. Figures for Gardner State Hospital, Massachusetts, were obtained from Annual Report of the Commissioner of Mental Diseases. Figures for Central State Hospital, Raleigh, North Carolina, were obtained from "Study of Mental Health, North Carolina." Figures for Milwaukee County Hospital were obtained from "Survey of Wisconsin" by Mental Hospital Survey Committee. All other figures for nursing personnel were obtained from "Report on Hospitalization of the Mentally Ill" (House of Delegates, A.M.A., June 1933).

up to the standard. More than twice the expected load is found in 24 hospitals which constitute 18 per cent of the total.

The regions with the lowest patient load per nurse and attendant are New England and the Middle Atlantic

GRAPH 3

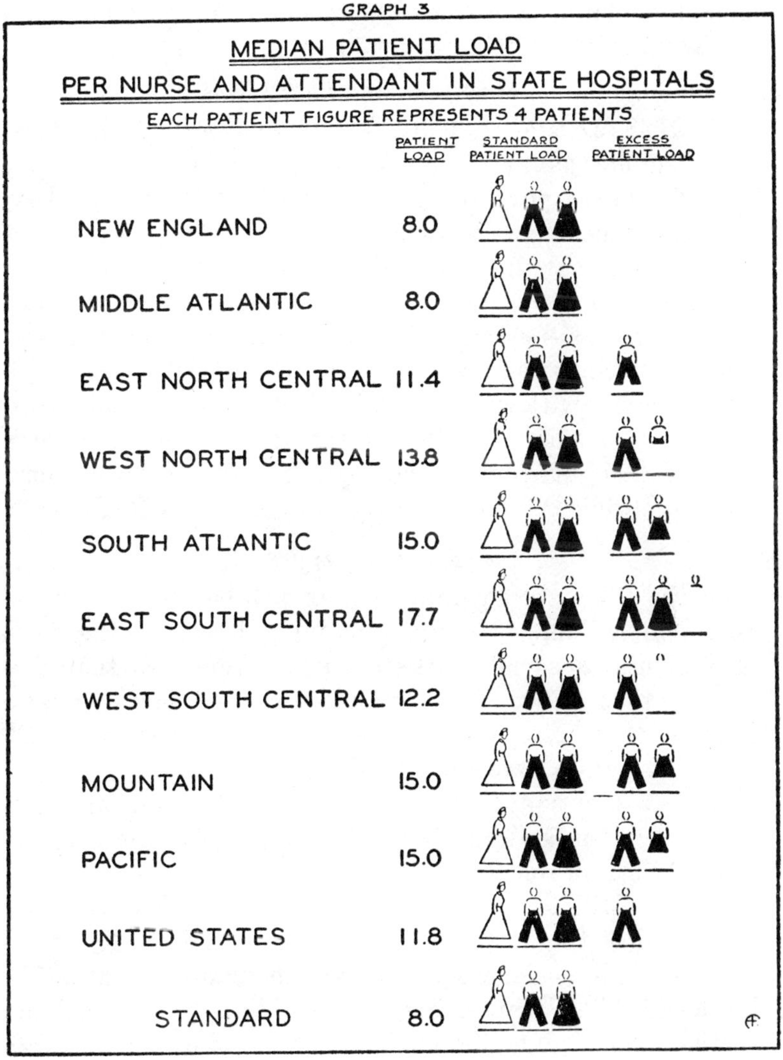

MEDIAN PATIENT LOAD
PER NURSE AND ATTENDANT IN STATE HOSPITALS
EACH PATIENT FIGURE REPRESENTS 4 PATIENTS

	PATIENT LOAD	STANDARD PATIENT LOAD	EXCESS PATIENT LOAD
NEW ENGLAND	8.0		
MIDDLE ATLANTIC	8.0		
EAST NORTH CENTRAL	11.4		
WEST NORTH CENTRAL	13.8		
SOUTH ATLANTIC	15.0		
EAST SOUTH CENTRAL	17.7		
WEST SOUTH CENTRAL	12.2		
MOUNTAIN	15.0		
PACIFIC	15.0		
UNITED STATES	11.8		
STANDARD	8.0		

Region, each with a median of less than eight. The East South Central Region has the highest patient load per nurse and attendant—17.7.

The patient load per nurse and attendant in the psychiatric and psychopathic hospitals was less than eight. For the Veterans Administration Facilities and the institutions for mental defectives and epileptics no adequate data were available.

3. Occupational Therapists

Of the 127 state hospitals, 13 per cent of the total reported not having any occupational therapists, 13 per cent did not respond to this item, while 101 reported having one or more occupational therapists. The adequacy of the occupational therapy staff was estimated by calculating the ratio of patients to occupational therapists. The distribution of the ratio of patients to occupational therapists by regions is shown in Table X.

The region with the highest load per occupational therapist in its median hospital is the Pacific Region with a load of 1,600 or more. The regions with the lowest load are the Middle Atlantic and the New England Regions.

4. Social Workers

Of the 127 state hospitals, 41, or 32.3 per cent, reported no social workers. In the remaining hospitals the ratio of patients to social workers varied from less than 200 to more than 1,600. Two hospitals reported having a ratio of less than 200 patients per social worker while 23 reported a ratio exceeding 1,600.

The distribution of the ratio of patients to social workers by regions and the weighted ratings for these ratios are shown in Table XI.

In the Middle Atlantic States and in New England nearly all of the hospitals have social workers. The ratio of patients to social workers in the median hospital is 775 in the Middle Atlantic States and 833 in New England. In the other regions the median ratio is in excess of 1,600.

TABLE X

RATIO OF PATIENTS TO OCCUPATIONAL THERAPISTS IN STATE HOSPITALS, BY REGIONS

	New England	Middle Atlantic	East North Central	West North Central	South Atlantic	East South Central	West South Central	Mountain	Pacific	Total	Weighted Ratings
1–200	4	6	1	2	2	1				16	2
201–400	4	9	12	1			1			27	2
401–600	3	6	6	2	2		3			22	1
601–800		1	2	3						6	1
801–1,000		1	1	2	1			1	1	6	1
1,001–1,200			1	1	1		1			4	0
1,201–1,400	1				1		1			3	0
1,401–1,600					1	1	1			3	0
1,601 and over			1	1	1	1		3	2	9	0
0			2	2	5	2	1		4	16	0
Not stated	1	6	3	3				2		15	*
Total	13	28	29	17	14	5	8	6	7	127	
Regional Medians	325	212.1	450	767.7	1,301	1,600		1,601	1,601	303	

* Regional Median.

TABLE XI

RATIO OF PATIENTS TO SOCIAL WORKERS IN STATE HOSPITALS, BY REGIONS

	New England	Middle Atlantic	East North Central	West North Central	South Atlantic	East South Central	West South Central	Mountain	Pacific	Total	Weighted Ratings
1–200	1	3	1		1					2	2
201–400	2	4	1							5	2
401–600	3	8	1							7	2
601–800	3	3	1							13	2
801–1,000	1	4	4	2	1		1			13	1
1,001–1,200		1	4						1	9	1
1,201–1,400	2	2	1	1			1	1	1	6	1
1,401–1,600		2	7	4	3				1	6	1
1,601 and over	1	1	9	8	9		3	5	4	23	0
0				2		5	3			41	0
Not stated										2	*
Total	13	28	29	17	14	5	8	6	7	127	
Median	833.3	775	1,600	1,600	1,600	0	1,600	1,600	1,600	1,601	

* Regional Median.

GRAPH 4

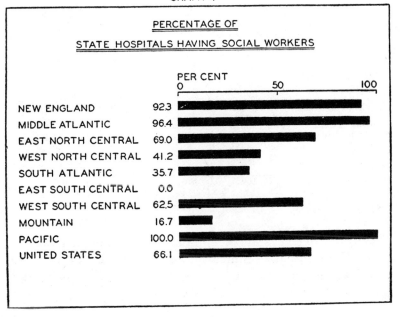

PERCENTAGE OF
STATE HOSPITALS HAVING SOCIAL WORKERS

	PER CENT
	0 50 100
NEW ENGLAND	92.3
MIDDLE ATLANTIC	96.4
EAST NORTH CENTRAL	69.0
WEST NORTH CENTRAL	41.2
SOUTH ATLANTIC	35.7
EAST SOUTH CENTRAL	0.0
WEST SOUTH CENTRAL	62.5
MOUNTAIN	16.7
PACIFIC	100.0
UNITED STATES	66.1

C. CLINICAL FACILITIES

The items included in this grouping consist of clinical directorship, clinical laboratory, percentage of deaths autopsied, out-patient clinics and medical library.

1. Clinical Director

The hospitals reporting this item varied in their responses considerably. These responses were classified according to the following five categories: 1, A specially designated clinical director devoting full time to supervision of the medical service; 2, A regular staff physician appointed to take care of this service; 3, The superintendent himself serving as clinical director; 4, No one performing the function of clinical director; 5, No response. The responses and the weights given to each of these categories are shown in Table XII.

TABLE XII

DISTRIBUTION OF CLINICAL DIRECTORS, BY TYPE

	State Hospitals		Psychopathic and Psychiatric Hospitals		Institutions for Mental Defectives and Epileptics		Veterans Administration Facilities		Weighted Ratings
	No.	Per cent	No.	Per cent	No.	Per cent	No.	Per cent	
Clinical Director..	32	25.2	7	63.7	3	5.7	5	21.7	3
Staff Physician....	29	22.8	4	36.3	23	43.4	18	78.3	2
Superintendent. ...	42	33.1	0		18	34.0	0		1
No Clinical Director	21	16.5	0		7	13.2	0		0
Not reported......	3	2.4	0		2	3.8	0		*
Total..........	127	100.	11	100.	53	100.	23	100.	
Median..........	1.98		2.21		1.02		2.64		

* Regional Median.

Only 32 of the state hospitals, or 25.2 per cent had a specially designated clinical director while 21, or 16.5 per cent had no one serving in this capacity. The remaining state hospitals had either the superintendent or a physician serving in that capacity.

In the psychiatric institutes and psychopathic hospitals all those reporting indicated that they had a clinical director and in only four of the hospitals did a regular staff physician occupy this position.

All of the Veterans Administration Facilities had some one designated as clinical director. A member of the staff gave full time to this work in only nine of these institutions, while in the remaining 18 or 78.3 per cent of these institutions, a regular staff member served in that capacity on a part-time basis.

In the institutions for mental defectives, there were only three, or 5.7 per cent that had clinical directors while seven, or 13.2 per cent reported no clinical director. The remaining institutions were divided equally between those in which the superintendent served as clinical director and those in which a staff member served in that capacity.

The weighted ratings shown in Table XII were applied

to the state hospitals in each region. The median rating
by regions is shown in Table XIII.

TABLE XIII

DISTRIBUTION OF MEDIAN RATINGS IN STATE HOSPITALS FOR TYPE OF CLINICAL
DIRECTOR, BY REGIONS

Region	Median
New England....................	1.1
Middle Atlantic.................	2.8
East North Central.............	1.0
West North Central.............	1.3
South Atlantic.................	1.7
East South Central.............	1.0
West South Central.............	1.2
Mountain......................	1.0
Pacific.......................	2.6
Total........................	1.5

The region with the highest median rating on this single
item was the Middle Atlantic Region, with a rating of
2.8, while the lowest rating was obtained by the East South
Central and the East North Central Regions, each with
a rating of 1.0.

2. *Laboratory Facilities*

All the institutions which responded to the question
regarding laboratory facilities indicated that they had

TABLE XIV

LABORATORY FACILITIES IN INSTITUTIONS FOR MENTAL DISEASE AND FOR
MENTAL DEFECT AND EPILEPSY

	State Hospitals		Psychopathic and Psychiatric Hospitals		Institutions for Mental Defectives and Epileptics		Veterans Administration Facilities		Weighted Ratings
	No.	Per cent	No.	Per cent	No.	Per cent	No.	Per cent	
Adequate Facilities. . . .	80	63.0	11	100.	25	47.1	22	95.6	2
Partially Adequate Facilities. . . .	29	22.9	0		13	24.5			1
Inadequate Facilities	17	13.4	0		14	26.4			0
Not stated.......	1	0.8	0		1	1.9	1	4.4	*
Total.	127	100.	11	100.	53	100.	23	100.	

* Regional Median.

some type of laboratory service. In some instances the laboratory facilities utilized were not in the hospital but in a neighboring medical school or central state laboratory. The laboratory service was reported as adequate, partially adequate or inadequate. The distribution of institutions by type of laboratory facilities is shown in Table XIV.

GRAPH 5

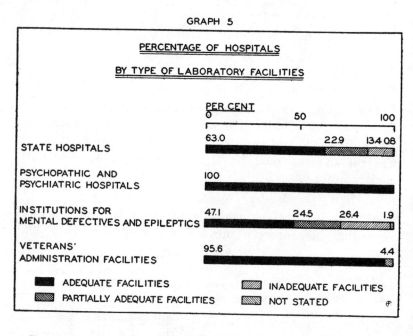

PERCENTAGE OF HOSPITALS

BY TYPE OF LABORATORY FACILITIES

PER CENT

STATE HOSPITALS

PSYCHOPATHIC AND PSYCHIATRIC HOSPITALS

INSTITUTIONS FOR MENTAL DEFECTIVES AND EPILEPTICS

VETERANS' ADMINISTRATION FACILITIES

ADEQUATE FACILITIES   INADEQUATE FACILITIES
PARTIALLY ADEQUATE FACILITIES   NOT STATED

In the state hospitals, 80, or 63 per cent of the total, reported having adequate facilities and 17, or 13.4 per cent reported having inadequate facilities. The remaining institutions reported having partially adequate facilities.

All the psychiatric and psychopathic hospitals reported adequate facilities.

In institutions for mental defectives 25 or 47.1 per cent of the total reported adequate facilities, 14 or 26.4 per cent reported inadequate facilities, and 13 or 24.5 per cent partially adequate facilities.

All but one of the Veterans Administration Facilities reported adequate facilities.

The distribution of the laboratory facilities in the state hospitals by regions on the basis of weighted ratings assigned to each type of laboratory facility indicates that the state hospitals in the Pacific Region had the highest median in laboratory facilities while the hospitals in the East South Central Region had the lowest rating. These data are shown in Table XV.

TABLE XV

DISTRIBUTION OF MEDIAN RATINGS FOR LABORATORY FACILITIES IN THE STATE HOSPITALS OF EACH REGION

Region	Ratings
New England	1.5
Middle Atlantic	1.8
East North Central	1.6
West North Central	1.8
South Atlantic	1.6
East South Central	0.8
West South Central	1.9
Mountain	1.0
Pacific	2.0
Total	1.7

3. Percentage of Deaths Autopsied

The item requesting information about the percentage of deaths autopsied yielded a large number of unknowns because of an error in the statement of the questionnaire. Thirty-five of the state hospitals, 12 of the institutions for mental defectives and a large proportion of the remaining institutions gave no information on this point. However, for the institutions for which information was available the percentage of deaths autopsied ranged from 0 to 100.

Nineteen of the state hospitals for mental disease reported that the percentage of deaths autopsied in their institutions was between 90 and 100 per cent, while 18 state hospitals reported no autopsies whatsoever. The median per cent of deaths autopsied for the state hospitals was 28.

In the psychiatric and psychopathic institutions there was a wide variation, with one hospital reporting no autopsies and one hospital reporting between 70 and 80 per cent of deaths autopsied.

In the institutions for mental defectives eight reported between 90 and 100 per cent of deaths autopsied, 19 reported no autopsies whatsoever, the median per cent of autopsies being 5 per cent.

In the Veterans Administration Facilities 5 reported 100 per cent of deaths autopsied, while 2 reported no autopsies.

The medians for some of the regions of the country are not very reliable since only a few hospitals reported, but for those institutions for which data were available the region with the highest percentage of autopsies was the East North Central. The region with the lowest was the South Atlantic, while the following regions—West South Central, Mountain and Pacific—did not have sufficient information to establish a median. (See Tables XVI and XVII.)

TABLE XVI

PERCENTAGE OF DEATHS AUTOPSIED IN INSTITUTIONS FOR MENTAL DISEASE AND FOR MENTAL DEFECT AND EPILEPSY

	State Hospitals		Psychopathic and Psychiatric Hospitals		Institutions for Mental Defectives and Epileptics		Veterans Administration Facilities	
	No.	Per cent	No.	Per cent	No.	Per cent	No.	Per cent
91–100........	19	15.0	0		8	15.1	5	21.8
81–90.........	0		0		0		2	8.7
71–80.........	0		1	9.1	0		1	4.4
61–70.........	2	1.6	1	9.1	0		3	13.0
51–60.........	7	5.5	1	9.1	1	1.9	0	
41–50.........	11	8.7	0		3	5.7	2	8.7
31–40.........	4	3.2	2	18.2	3	5.7	2	8.7
21–30.........	13	10.2	2	18.2	6	11.3	0	
11–20.........	14	11.0	0		0		0	
Under 10........	4	3.2	0		1	1.9	0	
0..............	19	14.2	1	9.1	19	35.8	2	8.7
Not stated.......	35	27.8	3	27.3	12	22.6	6	26.1
Total.........	127	100.	11	100.	53	100.	23	100.
Median.........	28		35		5		68	

TABLE XVII

PERCENTAGE OF DEATHS AUTOPSIED IN STATE HOSPITALS, BY REGIONS

Percentage	New England	Middle Atlantic	East North Central	West North Central	South Atlantic	East South Central	West South Central	Mountain	Pacific	Total
91–100	1	4	5	4	1	1	2	1	0	19
81–90	0	0	0	0	0	0	0	0	0	0
71–80	0	0	0	0	0	0	0	0	0	0
61–70	0	0	0	1	0	0	0	0	1	2
51–60	1	1	4	1	0	0	0	0	0	7
41–50	2	6	2	0	1	0	0	0	0	11
31–40	0	1	0	2	0	0	0	1	0	4
21–30	2	5	2	0	3	0	0	0	1	13
11–20	2	7	3	2	0	0	0	0	0	14
Under 10	1	2	1	0	0	0	0	0	0	4
0	1	0	2	3	3	3	2	2	1	17
Not stated	3	2	10	4	6	1	4	2	4	36
Total	13	28	29	17	14	5	8	6	7	127
Median	25	28	48	37	23	*	*	*	*	281

* Indeterminate because of small number of cases.

4. Out-Patient Clinics

The responses to the question on out-patient clinics were categorized as follows: having regular out-patient clinics; occasional out-patient clinics; no out-patient clinics; and unknown.

Of the 127 state hospitals, 62 or 48.8 per cent reported having out-patient clinics, while 39 or 30.7 per cent reported no such clinic, and 23 reported occasional clinics. Of the 11 psychiatric hospitals, 9 reported having clinics, one reported no clinic and one reported an occasional clinic. In the 23 Veterans Administration Facilities, 12 reported having clinics, 7 having no clinics and 4 an occational clinic. Of the 53 institutions for mental defectives, 16 or 30.2 per cent reported having clinics, 26 or 49.1 per cent reported not having clinics, and 8 or 15.1 per cent reported having an occasional clinic.

When the median ratings for the item on clinics in the state hospitals were computed by regions, the highest

TABLE XVIII

OUT-PATIENT CLINICS IN INSTITUTIONS FOR MENTAL DISEASE AND FOR MENTAL DEFECT AND EPILEPSY

	State Hospitals		Psychopathic and Psychiatric Hospitals		Institutions for Mental Defectives and Epileptics		Veterans Administration Facilities		Total		Weighted Ratings
	No.	Per cent	No.	Per cent	No.	Per cent	No.	Per cent	No.	Per cent	
Have Clinics	62	48.8	9	81.8	16	30.2	12	52.2	99	46.3	2
Occasional Clinic	23	18.1	1	9.1	8	15.1	4	17.4	36	16.8	1
No Clinics	39	30.7	1	9.1	26	49.1	7	30.4	73	34.1	0
Not Reported	3	2.4	0		3	5.7	0		6	2.8	*
Total	127	100.	11	100.	53	100.	23	100.	214	100.	

* Regional Median.

median ratings were found for the Middle Atlantic and
the New England States, while the East South Central
States obtained the lowest rating. (See Table XVIII
and XIX.)

TABLE XIX

MEDIAN RATINGS FOR OUT-PATIENT CLINICS IN THE STATE HOSPITALS
OF EACH REGION

Region	Ratings
New England	1.8
Middle Atlantic	1.9
East North Central	1.6
West North Central	0.3
South Atlantic	0.5
East South Central	0.0
West South Central	0.3
Mountain	0.3
Pacific	1.6
Total	1.5

GRAPH 6

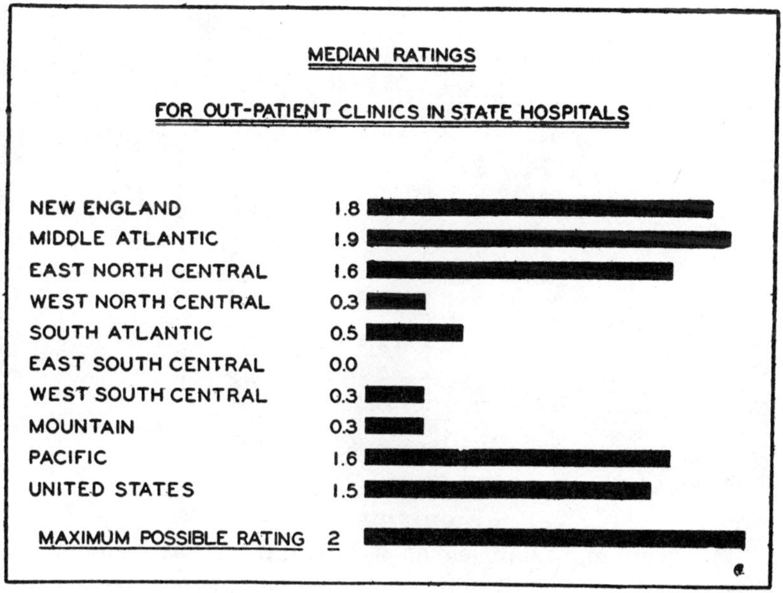

MEDIAN RATINGS

FOR OUT-PATIENT CLINICS IN STATE HOSPITALS

NEW ENGLAND	1.8
MIDDLE ATLANTIC	1.9
EAST NORTH CENTRAL	1.6
WEST NORTH CENTRAL	0.3
SOUTH ATLANTIC	0.5
EAST SOUTH CENTRAL	0.0
WEST SOUTH CENTRAL	0.3
MOUNTAIN	0.3
PACIFIC	1.6
UNITED STATES	1.5
MAXIMUM POSSIBLE RATING	2

5. Medical Library

Data were obtained on several aspects of the library—
number of books, amount spent annually and number of
journals. The best single index of library adequacy was

the number of periodicals received in the library. This measure differentiated between the "good" and the "poor" institutions. The range in number of medical journals was from 0 to 33. The median state hospital had 10 journals in its medical library while 6 institutions reported no journals and 3 institutions reported as many as 33. In the Veterans Administration Facilities the median was 18.5 journals. In the institutions for mental defectives the median institution had 8.2 journals while 4 had no journals at all and 2 had as many as 33.

TABLE XX

NUMBER OF JOURNALS IN LIBRARIES OF INSTITUTIONS FOR MENTAL DISEASE AND FOR MENTAL DEFECT AND EPILEPSY

	State Hospitals		Psychopathic and Psychiatric Hospitals		Institutions for Mental Defectives and Epileptics		Veterans Administration Facilities		Weighted Ratings
	No.	Per cent	No.	Per cent	No.	Per cent	No.	Per cent	
31–33	3	2.4	0		2	3.8	1	4.4	3
28–30	1	0.8	0		1	1.9	1	4.4	3
25–27	4	3.2	0		1	1.9	1	4.4	3
22–24	2	1.6	0		0	9.0	2	8.7	3
19–21	7	5.5	1	9.1	2	3.6	3	13.0	2
16–18	8	6.3	0		2	3.8	5	21.8	2
13–15	8	6.3	0		6	11.3	2	8.7	2
10–12	17	13.4	2	18.2	5	9.4	0		1
7–9	15	11.8	0		6	11.3	0		1
4–6	23	18.1	1	9.1	8	15.1	0		1
1–3	6	4.7	0		6	11.3	0		0
0	6	4.7	0		4	7.5	0		0
Not stated	27	21.2	6	54.6	10	18.9	8	34.8	*
Total	127	100.	11	100.	53	100.	23	100.	
Median	10.0		11.2		8.2		18.5		

* Regional Median.

D. TEACHING FACILITIES

The teaching facilities of a hospital are an important factor in its research activities. Hospitals that are teaching centers attract able men and permit younger men to learn from their masters. In this manner they are not only contributing directly in furthering science, but indirectly in training more men. The items dealing with training facilities consist of: internes and their proportion to the total staff; supervision of internes; junior medical staff and its proportion to the total staff; and rotation of service.

The ratio of internes to the total staff proved to be a good item for differentiating the "better" from the "poorer" research hospitals. In the 32 poorer hospitals, the average percentage that internes constituted of the total staff was 0.43 per cent, while in the 32 better hospitals the average percentage was 11.7 per cent. For this reason this item was included in the total rating. The junior medical staff constituted 0.75 per cent of the total staff in the "poor" hospitals and 27.7 per cent of the total staff in the "good" hospitals. This item, too, was included in the total rating.

1a. Number of Internes

In 72 state hospitals, constituting 56.8 per cent of the total, no internes were reported. In the other hospitals the internes constituted from 1 to 75 per cent of the total medical staff. Table XXI shows the distribution of the percentage of internes to the total medical staff. The median percentage of internes on the staffs of state hospitals is 1 per cent.

TABLE XXI

PROPORTION OF INTERNES ON MEDICAL STAFF IN STATE HOSPITALS
FOR MENTAL DISEASE

Percentages	State Hospitals		Weighted Ratings
	No.	Per cent	
51–75.	2	1.6	3
26–50.	17	13.4	2
1–25.	36	28.4	1
0.	62	48.9	0
Not stated.	10	7.9	*
Total.	127	100.	

* Regional Median.

1b. Supervision of Internes

The supervision of the internes was rated on a three step-scale—no supervision, fair supervision, and good active supervision. The distribution of internes by type of supervision is shown in Table XXII.

TABLE XXII

Distribution of Internes, by Type of Supervision

	State Hospitals		Weighted Ratings
	No.	Per cent	
Good—Active.............	53	41.7	2
Fair.....................	2	1.6	1
None....................	0	0.0	0
No internes or no response...	72	56.8	*
Total...................	127	100.	

* Regional Median.

Only two hospitals were rated as having only fair super-vision and 53 as having good active supervision. No hospital in which there were internes was reported as having no supervision.

2. *Junior Medical Staff*

The junior medical staff constituted from 0 to 100 per cent of the total medical staff. The distribution is shown in Table XXIII.

TABLE XXIII

Proportion of Junior Medical Staff to Total Medical Staff

Percentages	State Hospitals		Weighted Ratings
	No.	Per cent	
61–100..................	10	7.9	3
31–60...................	18	14.2	2
1–30....................	53	41.7	1
0.......................	24	18.9	0
Not stated...............	22	17.3	*
Total...................	127	100.	

* Regional Median.

In 46 state hospitals, constituting 36 per cent of the total number of state hospitals, there were no junior medical officers. In the 83 remaining hospitals the junior medical staff constituted from 1 to 100 per cent of the total staff.

3. *Rotation of Service*

The value of the training that the internes and junior members of the medical staff receive depends on the extent to which the men on the various services are rotated. In Table XXIV the number of state hospitals having internes and other junior medical officers as well as the number having rotation of service is shown.

TABLE XXIV

ROTATION OF SERVICE OF JUNIOR MEDICAL STAFF AND INTERNE STAFF
IN STATE HOSPITALS FOR MENTAL DISEASE

Region	Hospitals * Without Junior Medical Staff and Internes	Hospitals With Rotation	Hospitals Without Rotation	Hospitals Not Reporting	Total
New England.	1	6	4	2	13
Middle Atlantic.	2	22	4		28
East North Central.	8	11	8	2	29
West North Central.	3	6	5	3	17
South Atlantic.	6	7	1		14
East South Central.	2	2	1		5
West South Central.	2	4	2		8
Mountain.	4	2			6
Pacific.		7			7
Total.	28	67	25	7	127

* Includes hospitals that had neither internes nor junior medical officers.

GRAPH 7

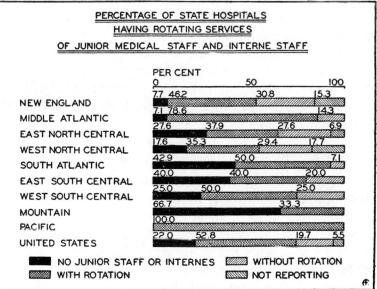

PERCENTAGE OF STATE HOSPITALS
HAVING ROTATING SERVICES
OF JUNIOR MEDICAL STAFF AND INTERNE STAFF

The responses to the item on rotation of service were classified as follows: having rotating service, partial rotating service, and no service. The weighted ratings for each of these responses were as follows:

Category	Weighted Ratings
Rotating service	2
Partial rotating service..........	1
No service.	0
Not stated.	Regional Median

Of the 127 state hospitals, 28, or 22 per cent, had no junior medical staff or internes. Of the remaining 99 hospitals, 67 had rotation of service, 25 did not have it, while 7 failed to report.

Nine of the 11 psychiatric institutes and psychopathic hospitals reported having a rotation of service.

In the Veterans Administration Facilities, 9 had rotating service and 9 reported that they had no internes or junior medical staff, while 2 had a partially rotating service.

In the institutions for mental defectives, 9, or 17 per cent, had a rotating service, while 32, or 60.4 per cent, had no internes or junior medical staff.

When the weighted ratings for this service were applied to the individual hospitals by regional areas, the region with the highest median rating was found to be the Middle Atlantic, the region with the lowest median rating the Mountain Region.

4a. University Contacts—Type of Contact

The responses to this item were classified under the following four headings: 1, Intimate contact with the university; 2, Occasional or little contact; 3, No contact; and 4, Unknown. The responses and the weighted ratings for these responses are shown in Table XXV.

In the state hospitals, 42, or 33.1 per cent, reported having university contacts while 54, or 42.5 per cent, reported

TABLE XXV

UNIVERSITY CONTACTS OF INSTITUTIONS FOR MENTAL DISEASE AND FOR MENTAL DEFECT AND EPILEPSY

	State Hospitals		Psychopathic and Psychiatric Hospitals		Institutions for Mental Defectives and Epileptics		Veterans Administration Facilities		Weighted Ratings
	No.	Per cent	No.	Percent	No.	Per cent	No.	Per cent	
Intimate contact	42	33.1	11	100.	14	26.4	5	21.8	2
Occasional or little contact	28	22.0	0		13	24.5	3	13.0	1
No contact	54	42.5	0		25	47.2	15	65.2	0
Not stated	3	2.4	0		1	1.9	0		*
Total	127	100.	11	100.	53	100.	23	100.	

* Regional Median.

having no such contacts. Twenty-eight, or 22.0 per cent, of the remaining hospitals reported having an occasional contact. Three hospitals did not report.

All the psychiatric and psychopathic hospitals reported having university contacts.

In the institutions for mental defectives only 14, or 26.4 per cent, reported having university contact, while 25, or 47.2 per cent, reported no such contact and 13, or 24.5 per cent, reported having occasional or little contact.

TABLE XXVI

MEDIAN RATINGS FOR UNIVERSITY CONTACTS IN THE STATE HOSPITALS
OF EACH REGION

Region	Ratings
New England	0.4
Middle Atlantic	0.5
East North Central	1.2
West North Central	1.3
South Atlantic	0.3
East South Central	0.3
West South Central	1.0
Mountain	0.8
Pacific	0.4
Total	0.8

In the Veterans Administration Facilities only 5, or 21.7 per cent, reported university contact, while 15, or 65.3 per cent, reported occasional or little contact.

In analyzing the results for the state hospitals it was found that when these responses were weighted as shown in Table XXVI giving the highest rating to intimate contact with the university and lowest to no contact, the region with the highest median rating for its hospitals was the West North Central Region with a rating of 1.3. The regions with the lowest rating were the East South Central and the South Atlantic, each with 0.3.

4b. Percentage of Hospital Staff on Medical School Faculties

The number of staff members who serve on the faculty of medical schools ranged from 1 to more than 3. The distribution is shown in Table XXVII.

TABLE XXVII

MEMBERS OF STATE HOSPITAL STAFF SERVING ON FACULTIES
OF MEDICAL SCHOOLS

Number of Faculty Members	State Hospitals		Weighted Ratings
	No.	Per cent	
3 and over.................	5	3.9	3
2.........................	8	6.3	2
1.........................	25	19.7	1
0.........................	76	59.7	0
Not stated.	13	10.2	*
Total...................	127	100.	

* Regional Median.

E. RESEARCH FACILITIES

The items dealing directly with research facilities are: number of staff members having research interests; type of research interest; and estimates of adequacy of general facilities for research exclusive of staff.

1. Percentage of Medical Staff Interested in Research

The range in the percentage of the medical staff having such interests was from 0 to 100 per cent. Eleven of the state hospitals, or 8.7 per cent, reported that more than 80 per cent of their staff had research interests, while 33, or 26 per cent, reported no members of their staff with such interests. In the psychiatric and psychopathic hospitals 5 of the hospitals reported staffs in which more than 80 per cent have research interests. In the Veterans Administration Facilities while one institution or 8.3 per cent of the total reported a staff in which 100 per cent of the members had interests in research, 9 institutions, or 39.2 per cent, reported no members with research interests.

In the institutions for mental defectives nine institutions or 4 per cent of the total reported that 90 per cent of their medical staff had research interests, while 20 institutions or 37.7 per cent reported no members with research interests.

The region with the highest median in the percentage of staff members with research interests was the West North Central with 32.7 per cent, while the region with the lowest was the Mountain Region with only 6 per cent. For the country as a whole the median hospital has 29.9 per cent of its medical staff interested in research. (See Tables XXVIII and XXIX.)

TABLE XXVIII

PERCENTAGE OF MEDICAL STAFF HAVING RESEARCH INTERESTS, BY TYPE OF INSTITUTION

Percentage	State Hospitals		Psychopathic and Psychiatric Hospitals		Institutions for Mental Defectives and Epileptics		Veterans Administration Facilities		Weighted Ratings
	No.	Per cent	No.	Per cent	No.	Per cent	No.	Per cent	
100.	9	7.1	4	36.4	9	17.0	1	4.4	9
91–99.	0		0		0		0		9
81–90.	1	0.8	1	9.1	0		0		9
71–80.	1	0.8	0		0		0		8
81–70.	3	2.4	0		1	1.9	0		7
51–60.	2	1.6	2	18.2	0		0		6
41–50.	8	6.3	0		4	7.6	1	4.4	5
31–40.	17	13.4	1	9.1	6	11.3	2	8.7	4
21–30.	18	14.2	2	18.2	3	5.7	2	8.7	3
11–20.	13	10.2	0		1	1.9	2	8.7	2
1–10.	7	5.5	0		0		3	13.1	1
0.	34	26.8	0		20	37.8	9	39.2	0
Not stated.	14	11.0	1	9.1	9	17.0	3	13.1	*
Total.	127	100.	11	100.	53	100.	23	100.	
Median.	22.4		60.0		23.3		3.3		

* Regional Median.

TABLE XXIX

PERCENTAGE OF MEDICAL STAFF IN STATE HOSPITALS HAVING RESEARCH INTERESTS, BY REGIONS

Percentage	New England	Middle Atlantic	East North Central	West North Central	South Atlantic	East South Central	West South Central	Mountain	Pacific	Total
81–100.	1	0	1	2	1	1	3	1	1	11
71–80.	0	1	0	0	0	0	0	0	0	1
61–70.	0	2	0	0	1	0	0	0	0	3
51–60.	1	0	1	0	0	0	0	0	0	2
41–50.	1	0	2	2	2	0	1	0	0	8
31–40.	2	4	5	3	1	1	0	0	1	17
21–30.	2	5	4	1	2	1	0	1	2	18
11–20.	1	7	2	1	1	0	0	1	0	13
1–10.	1	4	2	0	0	0	0	0	0	7
0.	3	3	7	4	5	2	4	3	2	33
Not stated.	1	2	5	4	1	0	0	0	1	14
Total.	13	28	29	17	14	5	8	6	7	127
Regional Median. . . .	26.0	19.6	23.5	32.7	23.5	26.0	21.0	6.0	26.0	22.9

GRAPH 8

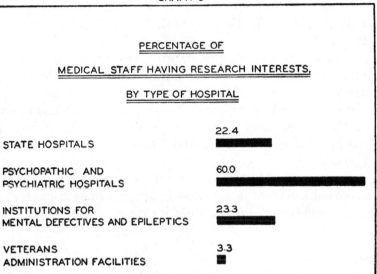

PERCENTAGE OF

MEDICAL STAFF HAVING RESEARCH INTERESTS,

BY TYPE OF HOSPITAL

STATE HOSPITALS   22.4

PSYCHOPATHIC AND   60.0
PSYCHIATRIC HOSPITALS

INSTITUTIONS FOR   23.3
MENTAL DEFECTIVES AND EPILEPTICS

VETERANS   3.3
ADMINISTRATION FACILITIES

GRAPH 9

PERCENTAGE OF MEDICAL STAFF IN STATE HOSPITALS

BY REGIONS

HAVING RESEARCH INTERESTS

MEDIAN PERCENTAGE

	0	50	100
NEW ENGLAND	26.0		
MIDDLE ATLANTIC	19.6		
EAST NORTH CENTRAL	23.5		
WEST NORTH CENTRAL	32.7		
SOUTH ATLANTIC	23.5		
EAST SOUTH CENTRAL	26.0		
WEST SOUTH CENTRAL	21.0		
MOUNTAIN	6.0		
PACIFIC	26.0		
UNITED STATES	22.9		

2. *Type of Research Interest*

Research interests were divided into two categories: Psychiatric and Neurological, and General Medical Research.

In the state hospitals 58, or 45.7 per cent, of the hospitals reported themselves as being interested in psychiatric or neurological research, while 34, or 26.8 per cent, of the hospitals reported no research interest whatsoever. Sixteen, or 12.6 per cent, of the total reported research interests in the general medical field, and 19, or 15 per cent, did not respond.

Ten of the 11 psychiatric and psychopathic hospitals reported interests in psychiatric and neurological research and the eleventh did not state its research interests.

TABLE XXX

MEDIAN RATINGS FOR TYPE OF RESEARCH INTEREST IN THE STATE HOSPITALS OF EACH REGION

Region	Ratings
New England	1.0
Middle Atlantic	1.9
East North Central	1.6
West North Central	1.5
South Atlantic	0.9
East South Central	1.0
West South Central	0.4
Mountain	0.3
Pacific	0.3
Total	1.6

In the Veterans Administration Facilities 9, or 39.1 per cent, of the hospitals reported having interests in the field of psychiatric and neurological research and 9, or 39.1 per cent, reported no research interests whatsoever.

In the institutions for mental defectives 15, or 28.3 per cent, reported themselves as having interests in psychiatric and neurological research while 21, or 39.6 per cent, reported no interests whatsoever and 7, or 13.2 per cent, reported interests in general medical research.

On the basis of the crude weighting of these items the region with the most adequate type of research interest

TABLE XXXI

TYPE OF RESEARCH INTEREST IN INSTITUTIONS FOR MENTAL DISEASE AND FOR MENTAL DEFECT AND EPILEPSY

	State Hospitals		Psychopathic and Psychiatric Hospitals		Institutions for Mental Defectives and Epileptics		Veterans Administration Facilities		Total		Weighted Ratings
	No.	Per cent	No.	Per cent	No.	Per cent	No.	Per cent	No.	Per cent	
Psychiatric and Neurological	58	45.7	10	91.0	15	28.3	9	39.1	92	43.0	2
General Medical	16	12.6			7	13.2	3	13.0	26	12.1	1
None	34	26.8			21	39.6	9	39.1	64	30.0	0
Not stated	19	15.0	1	9.1	10	18.9	2	8.7	32	15.0	*
Total	127	100.	11	100.	53	100.	23	100.	214	100.	

* Regional Median.

from the point of view of psychiatry was the Middle Atlantic with a rating of 1.9. The rating for research interest in the Pacific and Mountain Regions was only 0.3. (See Tables XXX and XXXI.)

3. Physical and Other Facilities for Research

The answers to the question regarding physical facilities for research were classified as follows:

Categories	Weights
Good	2
Fair	1
None	0
Unknown	Regional Median

This question aimed to determine what facilities, exclusive of personnel, were available in the institutions.

TABLE XXXII

MEDIAN RATINGS FOR PHYSICAL FACILITIES FOR RESEARCH IN THE STATE HOSPITALS, BY REGIONS

Region	Ratings
New England	0.8
Middle Atlantic	1.7
East North Central	1.5
West North Central	1.2
South Atlantic	1.0
East South Central	0.5
West South Central	1.0
Mountain	0.5
Pacific	1.3
Total	1.3

Fifty-one of the state hospitals, or 40.2 per cent of the total, reported having good facilities for research, 30, or 23.6 per cent, reported no facilities, and 31, or 24.4 per cent, reported fair facilities, while 15 or 11.8 per cent did not respond.

On the basis of the crude weights the region with the best research facilities was the Middle Atlantic while the regions with the poorest facilities were the East South Central and the Mountain Regions.

4. Number of Publications During the Last Three Years

The net result of the research in an institution usually appears in the form of a printed report either in scientific journals, monographs or books. There are, of course, many researches of a tentative kind that never appear in publication, but discounting these, the number of published reports may serve as a tentative gauge of the results of the research work. The number of publications together with the weighted ratings are shown in Table XXXIII.

TABLE XXXIII

NUMBER OF RESEARCH PUBLICATIONS DURING THE LAST THREE YEARS FROM THE STATE HOSPITALS

	New England	Middle Atlantic	East North Central	West North Central	South Atlantic	East South Central	West South Central	Mountain	Pacific	Total	Weighted Ratings
60		1								1	3
33–36		1								1	3
29–32										0	3
25–28		1								1	3
21–24		1								1	3
17–20										0	3
13–16		2								2	3
9–12		4	1							5	3
4–8	3	4	3	3						13	2
1–3	1	7	5	1	4		1	1		20	1
0	6	2	13	8	8	5	5	4	5	56	0
Unknown	3	5	7	5	2		2	1	2	27	*
Total	13	28	29	17	14	5	8	6	7	127	
Median	0.9	6	0.9	0.8	0.8	0	0.5	0.6	0	0.9	

* Regional Median.

From 56 state hospitals or nearly 50 per cent of the total not a single publication has appeared during the past three years. In 44 others, the number of publications varied from 1 to 60. The median number of publications was about 1 per hospital. The region with the highest number of publications was the Middle Atlantic with a median of 6 publications per hospital while from the East South Central and Pacific Regions no publications were reported during the past three years.

INDEX TO TABLES AND GRAPHS

PART V

APPENDICES

APPENDIX "A"

CODING FOR WEIGHTED RATINGS
(State Hospitals only—19 Items—Maximum Score: 66)

Wherever data were unavailable for determining the weighted rating of an item, the regional median for this item was used.

1. Number of Patients per Physician   Code number

Under 150	9
151–220	8
221–290	7
291–360	6
361–430	5
431–500	4
501–570	3
571–640	2
641–710	1
711 plus	0

2. Number of Patients per Nurse

Under 8	9
9–12	8
13–16	7
17–20	6
21–24	5
25–28	4
29–50	3
51–200	2
201–300	1
301–351 plus	0

3. Clinical Director

Special Clinical Director	3
Staff Physician	2
Superintendent or Assistant Superintendent	1
No Clinical Director	0

4. University Contact

Good	2
Occasional	1
None	0

5. Laboratory Facilities

Good	2
Fair	1
None	0

6. Percentage of Deaths Autopsied   Code number

         91–100................................   3

         31–90.................................   2

         11–30.................................   1

         0–10.................................   0

7. Out-patient Service

         Regular Service....................   2

         Partial Service.....................   1

         No Out-Patient Service...............   0

8. Rotating Service

         Regular........................   2

         Partial...........................   1

         None..........................   0

9. Number of Medical Journals

         22–33 plus........................   3

         13–21.............................   2

         4–12..............................   1

         0–3...............................   0

10. Percentage of Medical Staff Having Research Interests

         81–100.............................   9

         71–80..............................   8

         61–70..............................   7

         51–60..............................   6

         41–50..............................   5

         31–40..............................   4

         21–30..............................   3

         11–20..............................   2

         1–10...............................   1

         0...................................   0

11. Type of Research Interest

         Neurological—Psychiatric.............   2

         Medical...........................   1

         None..........................   0

12. Facilities for Research

         Good.............................   2

         Partial (Fair)......................   1

         None..........................   0

13. Number of Publications

         9–60...............................   3

         4–8................................   2

         1–3................................   1

         0..................................   0

14. **Number of Patients Per Occupational Therapist**   Code number

    1–400.   2

    401–1000.   1

    1001–plus (including no therapists)   0

15. **Number of Patients Per Social Worker**

    1–800.   2

    801–1600.   1

    1601 plus (including no social worker). .   0

16. **Ratio of Internes to Total Medical Staff**

    .51–.75.   3

    .26–.50.   2

    .10–.25.   0

    0.   0

17. **Supervision of Internes**

    Good—Active.   2

    Fair.   1

    None.   0

18. **Percentage of Junior Medical Staff to**
Total Medical Staff

    61.–100.   3

    31.–60.   2

    1–30.   1

    0.   0

19. **Members of Staff on Faculty**

    3 plus.   3

    2.   2

    1.   1

    None.   0

APPENDIX "B"

REGIONAL GROUPING OF STATES

New England
Maine
New Hampshire
Vermont
Massachusetts
Rhode Island
Connecticut

Middle Atlantic
New York
New Jersey
Pennsylvania

East North Central
Ohio
Indiana
Illinois
Michigan
Wisconsin

West North Central
Minnesota
Iowa
Missouri
North Dakota
South Dakota
Nebraska
Kansas

South Atlantic
Delaware
Maryland
District of Columbia
Virginia

South Atlantic—continued
West Virginia
North Carolina
South Carolina
Georgia
Florida

East South Central
Kentucky
Tennessee
Alabama
Mississippi

West South Central
Louisiana
Oklahoma
Texas
Arkansas

Mountain
Montana
Idaho
Wyoming
Colorado
New Mexico
Utah
Nevada
Arizona

Pacific
Washington
Oregon
California

APPENDIX " C "

INSTITUTIONS SURVEYED

State Hospitals for Mental Disease *

New England

Maine   Augusta State Hospital, Augusta
                        Bangor State Hospital, Bangor

New Hampshire   New Hampshire State Hospital, Concord

Vermont   Vermont State Hospital, Waterbury

Massachusetts   Westborough State Hospital, Westborough
                        Foxborough State Hospital, Foxborough
                        Bridgewater State Hospital, Bridgewater
                        Gardner State Hospital, East Gardner
                        Medfield State Hospital, Harding
                        Grafton State Hospital, North Grafton
                        Taunton State Hospital, Taunton
                    **Boston State Hospital, Boston
                    **Worcester State Hospital, Worcester

Connecticut   Fairfield State Hospital, Newtown
                        Norwich State Hospital, Norwich

Middle Atlantic

New Jersey   New Jersey State Hospital, Greystone Park
                        New Jersey State Hospital, Marlboro
                        Trenton State Hospital, Trenton

* Including 3 County and City Hospitals.
** Included in write-up of research centers but not in statistical evaluation.

Pennsylvania

Warren State Hospital, Warren
Danville State Hospital, Danville
Farview State Hospital, Waymart
Wernersville State Hospital, Wernersville
Norristown State Hospital, Norristown
Allentown State Hospital, Allentown
Harrisburg State Hospital, Harrisburg

New York

Binghamton State Hospital, Binghamton
Brooklyn State Hospital, Brooklyn
Buffalo State Hospital, Buffalo
Central Islip State Hospital, Central Islip
Creedmoor State Hospital, Queens Village
Gowanda State Homeopathic Hospital, Helmuth
Harlem Valley State Hospital, Wingdale
Hudson River State Hospital, Poughkeepsie
Kings Park State Hospital, Kings Park
Manhattan State Hospital, New York City
Marcy State Hospital, Marcy
Middletown State Homeopathic Hospital, Middletown
Pilgrim State Hospital, Brentwood
Rochester State Hospital, Rochester
Rockland State Hospital, Orangeburg
St. Lawrence State Hospital, Ogdensburg
Utica State Hospital, Utica
Willard State Hospital, Willard

East North Central

Michigan

Ypsilanti State Hospital, Ypsilanti
Ionia State Hospital, Ionia
Kalamazoo State Hospital, Kalamazoo
Newberry State Hospital, Newberry
Pontiac State Hospital, Pontiac
Traverse City State Hospital, Traverse City
Wayne County Hospital, Eloise

Ohio

Masillon State Hospital, Masillon
Cleveland State Hospital, Cleveland
Toledo State Hospital, Toledo
Dayton State Hospital, Dayton
Athens State Hospital, Athens
Columbus State Hospital, Columbus
Longview State Hospital, Longview
Lima State Hospital, Lima

Indiana	Central State Hospital, Indianapolis
	Logansport State Hospital, Longcliff
	Madison State Hospital, North Madison
	Richmond State Hospital, Richmond
Illinois	Manteno State Hospital, Manteno
	Peoria State Hospital, Peoria
	Chicago State Hospital, Chicago
	Elgin State Hospital, Elgin
	Alton State Hospital, Alton
	East Moline State Hospital, East Moline
	Kankakee State Hospital, Kankakee
Wisconsin	Northern Hospital for Insane, Winnebago
	Central State Hospital, Waupun
	Milwaukee County Hospital, Milwaukee

West North Central

Minnesota	Fergus Falls State Hospital, Fergus Falls
	Anoka State Asylum, Anoka
	Rochester State Hospital, Rochester
	Willmar State Asylum, Willmar
Iowa	Independence State Hospital, Independence
Missouri	State Hospital No. 1, Fulton
	State Hospital No. 2, St. Joseph
	State Hospital No. 3, Nevada
	State Hospital No. 4, Farmington
	St. Louis City Sanitarium, St. Louis
North Dakota	North Dakota State Hospital, Jamestown
South Dakota	Yankton State Hospital, Yankton

Nebraska

Hastings State Hospital, Ingleside
Lincoln State Hospital, Lincoln
Norfolk State Hospital, Norfolk

Kansas

Larned State Hospital, Larned
Topeka State Hospital, Topeka

South Atlantic

Virginia

Southwestern State Hospital, Marion
Western State Hospital, Staunton
Central State Hospital, Petersburg
Eastern State Hospital, Williamsburg

Delaware

Delaware State Hospital, Farnhurst

Maryland

Spring Grove State Hospital, Catonsville
Eastern Shore State Hospital, Cambridge
Springfield State Hospital, Sykesville

North Carolina

Goldsboro State Hospital, Goldsboro
Central State Hospital, Raleigh

Florida

Florida State Hospital, Chattahoochee

West Virginia

Huntington State Hospital, Huntington
Lakin State Hospital, Lakin
Weston State Hospital, Weston

East South Central

Tennessee

Eastern State Hospital, Knoxville
Western State Hospital, Bolivar
Central State Hospital, Nashville

Kentucky   Western State Hospital, Hopkinsville
Central State Hospital, Lakeland

West South Central

Oklahoma   Western Oklahoma State Hospital, Supply
Central State Hospital, Norman

Arkansas   State Hospital, Little Rock

Louisiana   East Louisiana State Hospital, Jackson
Central Louisiana State Hospital, Pineville

Texas   Rusk State Hospital, Rusk
Wichita Falls State Hospital, Wichita Falls
San Antonio State Hospital, San Antonio

Mountain

Colorado   Colorado State Hospital, Pueblo

New Mexico   New Mexico State Hospital, Las Vegas

Utah   Utah State Hospital, Provo

Wyoming   Wyoming State Hospital, Evanston

Idaho   State Hospital South, Blackfoot
State Hospital North, Orofino

Pacific

California   Agnews State Hospital, Agnews
                  Mendocino State Hospital, Talmage
                  Norwalk State Hospital, Norwalk
                  Patton State Hospital, Patton

Oregon   Oregon State Hospital, Salem
                  Eastern Oregon State Hospital, Pendleton

Washington   Northern State Hospital, Sedro Wooley
                  Eastern State Hospital, Medical Lake

State Institutions for Mental Defectives and Epileptics

New England

Maine   Pownal State School, West Pownal

New Hampshire   Laconia State School, Laconia

Vermont   Brandon State School, Brandon

Massachusetts   Monson State Hospital, Palmer
                  Belchertown State School, Belchertown
                  Walter E. Fernald State School, Waverley
                  *Wrentham State School, Wrentham

Rhode Island   Exeter School, LaFayette

Connecticut   Mansfield State Training School, Mansfield Depot

* Included in write-up of research centers but not in statistical evaluation.

Middle Atlantic

New Jersey

New Jersey State Village for Epileptics, Skillman
North Jersey Training School, Totowa
Woodbine Colony for Feebleminded Males, Woodbine
Vineland State Training School, Vineland

Pennsylvania

Polk State School, Polk
Laurelton State Village, Laurelton

New York

Albion State Training School, Orleans
Institution for Male Defective Delinquents, Napanoch
Newark State School, Newark
Wassaic State School, Wassaic
Craig Colony, Sonyea
Rome State School, Rome
Syracuse State School, Syracuse
Letchworth Village, Thiells

East North Central

Michigan

Wayne County Training School, Northville
Michigan Home and Training School, Lapeer
Michigan Farm Colony for Epileptics, Wahjamega

Ohio

Institution for Feebleminded, Columbus
Institution for Feebleminded, Orient

Illinois

Lincoln State School and Colony, Lincoln
Dixon State Hospital, Dixon

Wisconsin

N. Wisconsin Colony and Training School, Chippewa
Falls
S. Wisconsin Colony and Training School, Union
Grove

West North Central

Minnesota
:   School for Feebleminded, Faribault
    Minnesota Colony for Epileptics, Cambridge

Iowa
:   Hospital for Epileptics and School for Feebleminded, Woodward
    Institution for Feebleminded Children, Glenwood

Missouri
:   Missouri State School for Feebleminded and Epileptics, Marshall

South Dakota
:   State School for Feebleminded, Redfield

Nebraska
:   Nebraska Institution for Feebleminded, Beatrice

Kansas
:   State Hospital for Epileptics, Parsons
    State Training School, Winfield

South Atlantic

Virginia
:   State Colony for Epileptics and Feebleminded, Colony

Maryland
:   Training School for Feebleminded, Annapolis
    Rosewood State Training School, Owings Mills

Florida
:   Florida Farm Colony, Gainesville

West Virginia
:   West Virginia Training School, St. Marys

Alabama
:   Partlow State School, Tuscaloosa

West South Central

Texas   Abilene State Hospital (Epileptics), Abilene
          Austin State School (Feebleminded), Austin

Mountain

New Mexico   Home and Training School, Las Lunas

Wyoming   Wyoming State Training School, Lander

Idaho   State School and Colony, Nampa

Pacific

California   Sonoma State Home, Eldridge

Oregon   Oregon Fairview Home, Salem

Psychiatric and Psychopathic Hospitals

New England

Massachusetts   Boston Psychopathic Hospital, Boston

Middle Atlantic

New York   Psychiatric Institute and Hospital, New York City
          Syracuse Psychopathic Hospital, Syracuse
          Psychiatric Division, Bellevue Hospital, New York City

East North Central

    Michigan   State Psychopathic Hospital, Ann Arbor

    Illinois   Illinois Research Hospital, Chicago
                                    Cook County Psychopathic Hospital, Chicago

    Wisconsin   Wisconsin Psychiatric Institute, Madison

West North Central

    Iowa   Iowa State Psychopathic Hospital, Iowa

West South Central

    Texas   Galveston State Psychopathic Hospital, Galveston

Mountain

    Colorado   State Psychopathic Hospital, Denver

Veterans Administration Facilities and Federal Hospitals

New England

    Massachusetts   Veterans Administration Facility, Bedford
                                      Veterans Administration Facility, Northampton

Middle Atlantic

    New Jersey   Veterans Administration Facility, Lyons

| Pennsylvania | Veterans Administration Facility, Coatesville |

| New York | Veterans Administration Facility, Canandaigua |
| | Veterans Administration Facility, Northport |

East North Central

| Michigan | Veterans Administration Facility, Camp Custer |

| Ohio | Veterans Administration Facility, Chillicothe |

| Indiana | Veterans Administration Facility, Marion |

| Illinois | Veterans Administration Facility, N. Chicago |
| | Veterans Administration Facility, Danville |

West North Central

| Iowa | Veterans Administration Facility, Knoxville |

South Atlantic

| Georgia | Veterans Administration Facility, Augusta |

| Maryland | Veterans Administration Facility, Perry Point |

| District of Columbia | St. Elizabeths Hospital, Washington, D. C. |

East South Central

  Kentucky   Veterans Administration Facility, Lexington

  Mississippi   Veterans Administration Facility, Gulfport

West South Central

  Texas   Veterans Administration Facility, Waco

  Arkansas   Veterans Administration Facility, North Little Rock

Mountain

  Colorado   Veterans Administration Facility, Fort Lyon

  Wyoming   Veterans Administration Facility, Sheridan

Pacific

  California   Veterans Administration Facility, Palo Alto

  Washington   Veterans Administration Facility, American Lake

APPENDIX " D " (I)

ORIENTATION STUDY OF STATE MENTAL HOSPITALS
(Outline for interview with hospital executives)

NAME............................... INTERVIEWED BY..........

AFFILIATION ....

I. Basic Information

1. Patient population

2. Percentage of overcrowding, if any

3. Number of admissions yearly

4. Medical resources and arrangements
    - (a) Number of medical personnel   Ratio to patients
    - (b) Is there a well qualified clinical director?
    - (c) A Neurologist on staff or available?
    - (d) Is outside consulting staff utilized?
    - (e) Is there intimate contact with a university teaching center?
    - (f) Are there arrangements for regular clinical conferences?

5. Nursing resources and arrangements
    - (a) Number of nursing personnel
      On chronic services what is ratio to patients
      On acute and infirmary services what is ratio
    - (b) Is there a training school for nurses?

6. Laboratory arrangements
    - (a) Facilities
    - (b) Pathologist
    - (c) Technicians
    - (d) Number of autopsies performed per annum

7. Occupational therapy
    - (a) Are there well-trained supervisors?
    - (b) Is there participation by medical and nursing staffs?
    - (c) Proportion of patients served

8. Social work arrangements
    - (a) Number of social workers employed
    - (b) Training qualifications for appointment
    - (c) Number of cases under supervision per annum

9. Out-patient Services
    What arrangements

10. Does superintendent appoint members of the medical, nursing and technical staffs?   Are appointments made with consideration for factors other than merit?

II. Information Regarding Training Facilities

1. Internes
   (a) Number trained each year
   (b) Type of supervision

2. Junior Medical Staff
   (a) Qualifications for appointment
       age   previous general hospital interneship
       demonstrated interest in psychiatry
   (b) Arrangements for training
       Is there a well-qualified clinical director in charge of training program?
       During the first two years' attachment to hospital staff, are there opportunities for contacts and responsibilities in the reception and other clinical services?   In out-patient clinics? In laboratory work?   In clinical research?   In regular clinical conferences?
       What are the drawbacks, if any, in hospital arrangements that interfere with the clinical training of psychiatrists?

3. Library
   (a) Does it contain recent standard texts?
   (b) Approximate number of current journals
   (c) Amount spent on each of above during past year
   (d) Extent of use
   (e) Is recent literature discussed at staff conferences?

III. Information Regarding Research

1. What staff members have research interests in a broad sense? (Case studies, therapeutics, child guidance, criminology, special psychobiological projects)

2. What is their training and experience? Is it suited for research?

3. How much time can they devote to research?

4. What facilities have they for their particular interests?

5. What funds have they to draw upon?

6. What reference library facilities have they?

7. What have they produced in the past three years (original work and publications)?

8. What is the attitude of your governing body (visitors, trustees, State Department)?

9. What projects would you encourage if you had funds, and how much would you require?

10. Can you influence your legislature in an appropriation for research?

11. Are your facilities for research being used by any outside groups?

12. Are any of the members of your staff on the faculties of medical schools or universities?

13. Do you feel that the prosecution of research in your hospital would quicken the scientific interest of your staff, and substantially improve the care and treatment of patients?

14. Give names of young men on staff showing particular promise in research?

IV. Attitude Toward Development of Research Program

1. Do you think the time is opportune to urge governors and legislatures to make better arrangements for the extension of psychiatric research?
   And would it be desirable to have a certain percentage of state appropriations to mental hospitals definitely assigned to research?

2. Should research undertakings in your state be centralized in one research institute, or is it advisable to develop a program wherein the various mental hospitals participate?

3. Do you consider it desirable to have a central state planning for research in mental hospitals? With the collaboration of a national agency?

4. Is close linkage between the mental hospital and the medical school in regard to research desirable? What are the possibilities in your hospital for developing such affiliation?

5. Do you consider the opportunities for reseach men amply attractive in your hospital system? If not, what would you suggest to remedy the situation?

ADDITIONAL COMMENTS:

APPENDIX " D " (2)
RESEARCH FACILITIES

Name of Hospital

1. Patient population:

2. Admissions yearly:

3. Nominal capacity:

4. Number of physicians in addition to superintendent:

5. Number of nursing personnel:

6. Who acts as clinical director?

7. What contact do you maintain with a university center?

8. Are laboratory facilities adequate?

9. Autopsies per annum:

10. Proportion of deaths autopsied:

11. Number of occupation therapy aides:

12. Number of social workers:

13. Is there out-patient service?

14. Number of internes yearly:

15. Type of s u p e r v i s i o n of internes:

16. Number of junior medical staff members:

17. Is there rotating service?

18. Library:
   Number of periodicals:
   Approximate n u m b e r of books:
   Amount spent annually on books:

19. What staff members have research interests?
   Names
   Interest

20. What facilities have they?

21. Number of members on college or university faculties:

22. Projects of interest and funds desired:

23. Original work and publications in past 3 years:

   (a bibliography would be appreciated)

24. Comments (Please use back of sheet if necessary):

Reported by:

Date:

APPENDIX "E"

BIOGRAPHICAL DATA

This questionnaire has been arranged so as to require a minimum of **your** time. All information that is available in the American Medical Directory has been omitted. (Use additional sheets if necessary)

Date.................

1. Name

2. Place of birth

3. Sex (underscore)   Male   Female

4. Marital status   Children (number)

5. Premedical education (Include only collegiate work previous to entering medical school. If premedical work was combined with medical, please state this fact.)

College	Years of Study		Degree	Year Awarded
	From	To		

6. Interneships (Do not include any positions of a permanent nature)

	Name of Hospital	Dates of Service	
		From	To
(1) General............................		....	....
(2) Psychiatric.........................		....	....
(3) Neurological........................		....	....
(4) Other..............................		....	....

7. Private Practice

	Location	Type *	Dates of Service	
			From	To
(1)...................	....	....	....
(2)...................	....	....	....
(3)...................	....	....	....

* General medicine, psychiatry, neurology, other.

8. Present position..................................
              (Please give official title)
      Hospital
      Date of appointment

9. How appointed: Direct   Civil Service   Competitive Examination

10. Duties of present position (Indicate whether they are of a general char-
                        acter, or whether they are limited to a spe-
                        cific function such as reception service,
                        pathology, X-ray, etc.)

11. Present allowances (Indicate what accommodations and services the hos-
                        pital furnishes free of charge)
    Do you live in the hospital? (encircle)   Yes   No
    If living alone in the hospital: Number of rooms not counting bathroom
    . . . .
        Are you receiving subsistence? (encircle)   Yes   No
        Are you receiving laundry? (encircle)   Yes   No
        Other allowances (specify)
    If living with family in hospital: Number of rooms not counting bath-
        room. . . . .
        Are you receiving subsistence? (encircle)   Yes   No
        Are you receiving laundry? (encircle)   Yes   No
        Other allowances (specify)
        Number in family. . . . .

12. Previous positions in hospital service
    Date of entrance into state hospital service as a permanent appointee
    . . . .
    How many years have you spent in hospital service up to present time?
    . . . .
    List of all positions in hospital service, excluding interneships, in chron-
        ological order:

			Date of Service	
Name of Hospital	Location	Rank	From	To
. . . .	. . . .	. . . .	. . . .	. . . .
. . . .	. . . .	. . . .	. . . .	. . . .
. . . .	. . . .	. . . .	. . . .	. . . .
. . . .	. . . .	. . . .	. . . .	. . . .

13. Number of years spent in preparation (including interneships, medical
                        school and undergraduate study). . . . .

14. Other fields of experience and service (excluding medical) and medical
    consultant appointments, etc.

		Date of Service	
Type	Location	From	To
(a).	. . . .	. . . .	. . . .
(b).	. . . .	. . . .	. . . .
(c).	. . . .	. . . .	. . . .

15. Postgraduate study

| Courses | Where taken | Dates of Study | | Remarks |
		From	To	
....	....	....	....	....
....	....	....	....	....
....	....	....	....	....
....	....	....	....	....

16. Publications
    Approximate number
    Type (underscore)
                        Clinical
                        Laboratory
                        Statistical
                        Philosophical
    (A bibliography would be appreciated)

17. Teaching experience in Medical Schools

| Position | Location | Subject taught | Dates of Service | |
			From	To
....	....	....	....	....
....	....	....	....	....

18. Non-medical degrees Ph.D., Sc.D., M.A., LL.D., A.B., B.S. (specify others) (underscore)

INDEX

A

Acid-base balance of blood and brain, 45

Administrative technics, 51

Adolescence, manic-depressive reaction in, 67

Adolescent girls, dramatic work with, 60

Affiliation, 9, 10, 19

Agenesis, cerebral frontal, 69

Alcohol
effects on human organism, 45
effects on reaction time, 46
tolerance in relation to drinking habits, 45–46

Alcoholic intoxication, acute psychiatric study of, 46

Alcoholics
vitamin B complex in chronic, 28
vitamin therapy, 60

Alcoholism, 32, 70
and vitamin deficiency, 68
brain changes in, 60
with reference to blood and urine studies, 28

Anaphylaxis, 67

Anthropometric measurements, 54

Anthropometry, Physical, 63

Anti-toxins, 58

Appel, Kenneth E., 4

Art, 60

Arteriosclerosis, 68

Arthritides, 28

Association motor, use in the psychoneuroses, 28

Autopsies, 97–99
percentage of deaths autopsied in institutions for mental disease and for mental defect and epilepsy (Table XVI), 98
percentage of deaths autopsied in state hospitals, by regions (Table XVII), 99

Auxology, 63

B

Bacteria, importance of the morphological type upon physiological function of, 67

Barbiturate intoxication, 72

Basilar artery, size in schizophrenic patients, 40

Behavior disorders
group music in treatment of, 60
in children, course in management of, 37

Behavior problems in children
congenital syphilis in relation to, 38
heart disease in relation to, 38

Bellevue Hospital, 21, 58–61

Benzedrine
in post-encephalitis and dementia praecox, 32
physiological effects, 47

Benzedrine sulfate
effect on gall-bladder, 47
effect on mood and fatigue, 47

Berger rhythm waves, 30

Beri-beri in pigeons, 47

Birth injuries, 53, 61

Blood
alcohol curves, 46
and brain, acid-base balance of, 45
and cerebrospinal fluid barrier, 41
and spinal fluid alcohol, studies of, 46
cerebrospinal fluid bromide ratio, 41
chemistry during insulin coma, 60
chemistry studies, 71
flow, velocity of, 45
sedimentation in dementia praecox, 69
studies of cases of delirium tremens, 44
sugar in manic states, 58

Boston City Hospital, 22

Boston Psychopathic Hospital, 21, 43–46

RESEARCH IN MENTAL HOSPITALS
STUDY NUMBER TWO

*A Survey of Psychiatric Research Activities, Facilities,
Interests and Interrelationships as They Exist Under
Non-Governmental Auspices in the United States*

Conducted by
The National Committee for Mental Hygiene, Inc.
1939-1941

GEORGE S. STEVENSON, M.D., *Medical Director*

Assisted by

PAUL O. KOMORA
Associate Secretary

CLARA BASSETT
Consultant in Psychiatric Social Work

Advisory Committee

Clarence O. Cheney, M.D., *Chairman*   Joseph E. Raycroft, M.D.
Kenneth E. Appel, M.D.   *H. Douglas Singer, M.D.
Karl M. Bowman, M.D.   William J. Tiffany, M.D.
Adolf Meyer, M.D.   C. Fred Williams, M.D.

Ex-Officio Members

Samuel W. Hamilton, M.D.
Clarence M. Hincks, M.D.
Nolan D. C. Lewis, M.D.
Arthur H. Ruggles, M.D.

* Deceased

THE NATIONAL COMMITTEE FOR MENTAL HYGIENE, INC.
1790 BROADWAY, NEW YORK, N. Y.

Copyright, 1942, by

THE NATIONAL COMMITTEE FOR MENTAL HYGIENE, Inc.

Printed in the United States of America by

BOYD PRINTING COMPANY, Inc., ALBANY, N. Y.

FOREWORD

EARLY in 1938 The National Committee for Mental Hygiene reported its findings in a survey of the research activities, facilities and possibilities of state hospitals and other tax-supported institutions for the mentally ill and defective.* This survey was designed to "clear the way" for further progress in dealing with a major medico-social problem that takes an enormous toll both of individual lives and of individual and community wealth, and that shows signs of becoming even more serious.

The magnitude of this problem was pointed out in terms of the great and ever-growing demand for hospital and clinic accommodations for the care and treatment of sufferers from mental and nervous disorders. It was shown that the population of mental hospitals is increasing year after year, that in spite of therapeutic advances patients are entering these institutions in larger numbers than they are going out, and that we are in a critical phase of a situation that must be dealt with more aggressively. It was evident that the policy of building more and more hospitals to meet future increases is an insufficient answer to the problem, and it was felt that, among other measures, the acceleration of psychiatric research, looking toward more effective programs of prevention and treatment, offers one hope of "finding a better way." Research in mental and nervous diseases has revealed its value in many, though limited, ways. Its value in coping with other ills of man has long been recognized and is beyond argument.

Unfortunately, government—state and national—has concerned itself more with interferences with the monetary interests of man than it has with his satisfactory living, though there are enough exceptions to this rule to reveal

* *Research in Mental Hospitals.* A Survey and Tentative Appraisal of Research Activities, Facilities and Possibilities in State Hospitals and Other Tax-Supported Institutions for the Mentally Ill and Defective in the United States. 1938. The National Committee for Mental Hygiene, New York. 151 pp.

the great power inherent in public effort. But the initial advance usually seems to come from those individuals or private agencies that can "follow a hunch" on a day's notice, using whatever means happen to be at hand, and that have again and again furnished a stimulus to public progress. And so it seemed appropriate to follow the study of research in public mental hospitals with a complementary study and report of all the rest of our psychiatric research facilities. The present report brings together information about most of the important research centers operating under private auspices.

While an attempt has been made to differentiate private from public facilities, in practice it is not always possible to draw a clear distinction between the two. Our state universities, for example, usually combine endowment and public appropriation. Again, many of the researches of public agencies are supported by grants from private sources, and there are collaborative projects conducted by public and private agencies that defy classification under either. A glance at the earlier report will readily show many such arrangements. Conversely, it was found that by trailing research through private agencies one is led to the doors of many public agencies. The titles of the two respective studies are, therefore, not to be thought of as being in any sense antithetical, but rather as indicating important avenues to facilities, activities and opportunities that have much in common.

It seemed neither necessary nor desirable, in the light of these facts, to adhere rigidly to the title in deciding what to include in this report. It seemed more important to include a public agency that warranted mention in a discussion of research, and that might have been omitted from the previous report, than to respect the framework as such, for the least value of either report will lie in the words "public" or "private." It is the reference to research, in whatever setting, that is crucial.

One fact became quickly apparent in the first study that is further emphasized by the second study, namely, that research is only to a limited degree the expression of an institution. Where it is so confined, it is apt to be excessively parochial. In a broader sense research is the expression of a community and its spirit, and the products of research can best be understood by appreciating the network of persons and agencies that make up the "complex." It is hence easier to report research by communities rather than by institutions, and such is the pattern of this report. But a just appreciation of these research "complexes" can be had only if it is realized that this pattern is still limited and that the research potentialities of any place or person are determined by the richness of this network that may stretch over communities, states or the continent, on the one hand, or be sequestered within a small part of an institution, on the other. This is not meant to minimize in any way the importance of the critical, imaginative and aggressive research leader himself as a factor in the "complex."

It is intended that this report convey to those who are interested in the financing, or the support, or the prosecution of psychiatric research, some leads as to where their ambitions may find better opportunities for realization. It describes how its findings were sorted out of a large potential field; it discusses the organization and functions of different types of research set-up; it tells brief but salient stories of a number of research "complexes" or communities, as well as of individual research centers, and it attempts an analysis of some of the things about hidden men that man seems to be inquisitive about. The principal facts and findings are presented and interpreted in the main body of the report. Supplementary data concerning the extent and the character of researches in progress, the financial means available for investigative activities, and the personnel engaged in such activities, are presented in appendix form.

We extend cordial thanks to the John and Mary R. Markle Foundation, which liberally financed both the present and the preceding study, thus making it possible to round out our picture of psychiatric research in the United

States. We are grateful also to the special committee which advised and assisted us in the survey, and to all those who gave generously of their busy hours to show and to explain their work and who have endowed this creature with spirit.

GEORGE S. STEVENSON, M.D.
Medical Director,
The National Committee for Mental Hygiene

TABLE OF CONTENTS

CHAPTER I
Introduction

RESEARCH has long been regarded as a basic factor in medical progress. The phenomenal achievements of the medical and sanitary sciences in the control and prevention of many of man's physical ailments would not have been possible without it. Scientific investigation is no less important in the realm of mental disorders, when we consider the great frequency of these disorders and their far-reaching human, social and economic consequences. The lag of scientific progress in this field in the past, as compared with other branches of medicine, and the reasons therefor, are a familiar story. With the recent advances in psychiatry, however, the outlook has changed, and the possibilities and promise of mental medicine are commanding the serious attention of the biological, psychological, social and other contributory sciences.

The report of the American Medical Association, in the March 28, 1942, issue of its Journal, shows an average daily census of all hospitals * of 1,087,039.** Of these, 603,179, or about 55 per cent, were patients in mental hospitals. This does not mean that within a year there are more cases of mental disorder. Obviously more acute conditions occupy beds for a briefer time, and there are, in the course of a year, many more admissions for major and minor physical ailments than for mental conditions. It means, however, that mental conditions fill more hospital beds, at any one time, than all other disabling diseases combined and that mental illness is a major economic and public health problem. Scientists and laymen are advocating the vigorous extension of psychiatric research as a means of modifying present trends and promoting measures of control and prevention.

In an attempt to appraise the present status of psychi-

* Includes institutions for mental defectives and for epileptics.
** Figures are for the year 1941.

atric research and to explore the possibilities of a more vigorous and systematic attack on mental and nervous disorders by scientific means, The National Committee for Mental Hygiene, in 1936, embarked on a national survey with the three-fold object of determining (a) the extent and nature of present investigative work in tax-supported mental hospitals; (b) the facilities and resources, actual or potential, that lend themselves to the conduct of such work; and (c) the steps that can be taken to develop research activities in these institutions. Our report of this study gave a fairly comprehensive view of the research situation in public institutions for the mentally ill, providing, in the words of the report, "a factual basis which will serve as a point of departure and orientation toward the further and more rapid development of research interest and activity in public mental hospitals."

Subsequently, the National Committee undertook a similar survey of research under private auspices. Whereas the first study was concerned with the research possibilities existing in centers of vast patient populations—the state hospital—the second study taps the very heart of medical research and the fountainhead of much of our psychiatric leadership—the private non-proprietary hospital. Progress through research, in certain directions at least, comes about only through a degree of daring. The private hospital is in no particular jeopardy from the crossfire of political sniping and can venture into experimentation at the dictates of valid scientific leads that are sometimes startling, albeit human and ethical. The enhancement of these values is one of the prospective profits of such a study. The medical school with an investigative interest in psychiatry offers an atmosphere within which the medical student may develop a larger professional stature. A by-product of this study is to show where such atmosphere exists. It should be of interest also to those who are concerned with research in other branches of medicine, provided it be realized that the problems of organs are the problems of the man who carries them and whom they serve.

CHAPTER II
Scope and Methods of Survey

THE scope of this study was much less easily definable than that of the earlier study of tax-supported hospitals. There are so many small institutions in the private field that it was no small task to draw up a list that would be in any way comprehensive. Moreover, such institutions often merge into the university on the one hand and into the general hospital on the other, in such a way as to make it practically impossible to avoid missing some important instances of research carried on under unexpected auspices. Again, the relationship between tax-supported hospitals and medical schools is often so close that important research may be missed in one because it has been identified with the other.

Every effort was made in the beginning to comb lists in order to find hospitals and other institutions that are dealing with mental problems under private auspices. It is expected that omissions will be discovered later. Such omissions must be considered in large part an expression of the difficulties inherent in a survey of this nature and thus to some extent unavoidable. All known sources of information were utilized, however, and every care was exercised to achieve a reasonably thorough canvass of the field, and we venture to hope that few, if any, important centers of research have been overlooked.

As a first step, some 613 institutions were sent a return postcard on which they were asked to indicate whether or not "research projects in the field of psychiatry or especially related to psychiatric problems are now being conducted under the auspices of the institution or under the direction of any member of the attending or consulting staff." These institutions were situated in 41 different states. Those who did not reply to this first inquiry were sent a second return postcard. Sixteen of these were returned undelivered. In all, 242 replies were received, 62 indicating that research was a part of the activities of the institution, 180 answering in the negative. On the supposition that institutions interested in research would wish to be represented in a report of this character—since research reflects creditably on an institution's clinical work —it is reasonable to assume that few of the 371 institutions that did not reply engage in significant scientific activity. On the other hand, there may be, and there probably are, some that prefer not to have their activities publicized. Some who are conducting creditable investigations may not have answered us because they had this narrower concept. Many clinicians over the years have reported contributions from their observations which are just as important as material that is now being turned out as research. A good many hospital clinicians are making valuable studies which they do not call research because of their conception that research means that a man shall be enclosed in a laboratory or some isolated place where he works alone, doing as he pleases without reference to his fellow workers or to the broad aspects of conducting a hospital and treating patients.

A similar return card was addressed to 68 medical schools, again followed by a second return card where no reply was received to the first inquiry. No replies were received to either card from 11 schools, and of the remainder, 17 replied in the negative, while 40 claimed that research was going on.

The 62 institutions and 40 medical schools were each written to again for preliminary information as to researches under way, the names of the persons responsible for or conducting the studies, and the sources of financial support for the projects. Forty institutions and 32 medical schools responded with the details requested or otherwise.

Of the 40 institutions, 3 changed to the "no research" status, while 17 presented small, informal projects and showed no established research record as an institution. Of the remaining 20, 13 were independent units of established research standing of greater or less extent, and 7 were identified as parts of a larger complex, associated with another institution or medical school.

Of the 32 medical schools that responded, 6 were given full consideration in the first report, and so will be included here, if at all, only when referred to as part of a complex of facilities. Two medical schools that did not report were included in the previous study by affiliation. There were thus 26 medical schools whose research activities are due for consideration in this second study.

A glance at these 26 medical schools and 20 hospitals by any one having broad knowledge of the field of psychiatric research would promptly show that there are other sources of well known scientific contributions not included in this group. Without endeavoring to discover the reasons for these gaps, steps were taken to fill them.

As a next step, a canvass was made of the psychiatric literature published in 1938 and 1939, in order to discover active research centers that had not been revealed in the previous canvass-by-correspondence. The following periodicals were reviewed:

American Journal of Orthopsychiatry
American Journal of Psychiatry
Archives of Neurology and Psychiatry
Diseases of the Nervous System
Journal of Nervous and Mental Disease
Mental Hygiene
Proceedings of the American Association on Mental Deficiency
Psychiatry: Journal of the Biology and Pathology of Interpersonal Relations
Psychiatric Quarterly
Psychoanalytic Quarterly
Psychoanalytic Review
Psychomatic Medicine

As a result of this canvass of the literature, 37 additional centers were listed as potential centers and these were asked for details of research. Of these, 31 responded with detail, evidencing serious investigative activity. These were added to the 46 centers previously listed as appropriate for a visit. In the course of our study two other research centers were identified, thus bringing the total number of centers to 79.

It was noted during this canvass that many reports came into the psychiatric literature from non-psychiatric centers, such as university departments of psychology, public schools, courts, children's institutions, social agencies, state departments of welfare, and from many individuals (especially psychoanalysts, who require no laboratories). All these conduct research pertinent to psychiatry and they should all be kept in mind in any total picture of research, even though they are not psychiatric research centers of the type included in the purview of this report.

The number and classification of research centers and adjunct facilities covered in the present report is as follows: 10 medical school centers, including 10 associated hospitals (described in Chapter V); 10 other complexes, comprising 40 centers, including 16 medical schools and 35 hospitals, clinics and other facilities associated with them or otherwise forming part of these complexes (described in Chapter VI); and 29 individual centers (described in Chapter VII); making a total of 100 facilities. These facilities are located in 39 cities and towns in 22 states and the District of Columbia, distributed as follows:

MEDICAL SCHOOL CENTERS

GEORGIA
  Augusta
    University of Georgia School of Medicine and University Hospital

MICHIGAN
  Detroit
    Wayne University and Eloise Hospital

MINNESOTA
  Minneapolis-St. Paul
    University of Minnesota and Minnesota General Hospital

NEBRASKA
Omaha
University of Nebraska Medical School
Douglas County Hospital
Bishop Clarkson Memorial Hospital

NEW YORK
Albany
Albany Hospital and Medical College

New York
New York Hospital—Cornell University Medical College
Payne Whitney Psychiatric Clinic
New York Hospital—Westchester Division, White Plains
New York Post Graduate Hospital and Medical School

Syracuse
Syracuse Psychopathic Hospital and Syracuse University

OREGON
Portland
University of Oregon Medical School

TENNESSEE
Nashville
Vanderbilt University School of Medicine

OTHER COMPLEXES

CALIFORNIA
San Francisco
Stanford University
University of California
Medical School
Institute of Child Welfare, Berkeley
California Department of Institutions, Sacramento

CONNECTICUT
New Haven
Yale University
Medical School
Clinic of Child Development
Institute of Human Relations
New Haven Hospital
Psychiatric Service in the Community

ILLINOIS
Chicago
University of Chicago
Division of Biological Sciences

Otho S. A. Sprague Memorial Institute
Orthogenic School
Northwestern University
Michael Reese Hospital
Loyola University
Cook County Psychopathic Hospital
Institute for Psychoanalysis

KENTUCKY
Louisville
University of Louisville

MARYLAND
Baltimore
Johns Hopkins University
Henry Phipps Psychiatric Clinic
Harriet Lane Home
School of Hygiene and Public Health

MASSACHUSETTS
Boston
Harvard Medical School
Massachusetts General Hospital
McLean Hospital, Waverley
Peter Bent Brigham Hospital
Boston City Hospital
Children's Hospital
Tufts College Medical School
Habit Clinic for Child Guidance
Beth Israel Hospital
Judge Baker Guidance Center

MISSOURI
St. Louis
Washington University

OHIO
Cincinnati
University of Cincinnati
Cincinnati General Hospital
Jewish Hospital
Child Guidance Home
May Institute for Medical Research
Children's Hospital
Longview State Hospital

Cleveland
Western Reserve University
City Hospital
Cleveland Guidance Center

PENNSYLVANIA
  Philadelphia
    University of Pennsylvania
      School of Medicine
      Graduate School of Medicine
    Pennsylvania Hospital
      Institute of the Pennsylvania Hospital
    Philadelphia General Hospital
    Jefferson Medical College
    Temple University School of Medicine
    Gladwyne Colony, Gladwyne
    Elwyn Training School, Elwyn
    Philadelphia Child Guidance Clinic

INDIVIDUAL CENTERS

CALIFORNIA
  San Francisco
    Mount Zion Hospital

DISTRICT OF COLUMBIA
  Washington
    United States Public Health Service
      Public Health Service Hospital, Lexington, Ky.
      Public Health Service Hospital, Fort Worth, Tex.
    Catholic University of America

ILLINOIS
  Chicago
    Institute of General Semantics

KANSAS
  Topeka
    Menninger Sanitarium and Clinic and Southard School

MARYLAND
  Baltimore
    Children's Rehabilitation Institute
  Rockville
    Chestnut Lodge Sanitarium
  Towson
    Sheppard and Enoch Pratt Hospital

MASSACHUSETTS
  Boston
    Massachusetts Department of Mental Health
    Supreme Council, 33rd Degree, Scottish Rite, Northern Masonic
      Jurisdiction

Stockbridge
Austen Fox Riggs Foundation, Inc.

MICHIGAN
Detroit
Henry Ford Hospital

MISSOURI
Kansas City
Neurological Hospital

NEW JERSEY
Vineland
Training School at Vineland

NEW YORK
Albany
New York State Department of Mental Hygiene

Katonah
Pinewood

New York
Committee for the Study of Sex Variants
Hillside Hospital, Queens
Jewish Board of Guardians
Lifwynn Foundation
Mt. Sinai Hospital
New York Infirmary for Women and Children
New York Vocational Adjustment Bureau for Girls

Ossining
Stony Lodge

RHODE ISLAND
Providence
Butler Hospital
Emma Pendleton Bradley Home, East Providence

VIRGINIA
Richmond
Tucker Hospital
Westbrook Sanitarium

WISCONSIN
Wauwatosa
Milwaukee Sanitarium

RESEARCH CENTERS DESCRIBED IN EARLIER REPORT *

COLORADO
Denver
Colorado Psychopathic Hospital and University of Colorado

DISTRICT OF COLUMBIA
Washington
St. Elizabeths Hospital and George Washington University

ILLINOIS
Chicago
Illinois Psychiatric Institute and University of Illinois
Institute for Juvenile Research

Elgin
Elgin State Hospital

INDIANA
Indianapolis
Central State Hospital and Indiana University

IOWA
Iowa City
Iowa State Psychopathic Hospital and University of Iowa

MARYLAND
Catonsville
Spring Grove State Hospital

MASSACHUSETTS
Boston
Boston Psychopathic Hospital
Boston State Hospital

Worcester
Worcester State Hospital

Wrentham
Wrentham State School

MICHIGAN
Ann Arbor
Neuropsychiatric Institute and University of Michigan

Northville
Wayne County Training School

Ypsilanti
Ypsilanti State Hospital

* *Research in Mental Hospitals.* A Survey and Tentative Appraisal of Research Activities, Facilities and Possibilities in State Hospitals and Other Tax-Supported Institutions for the Mentally Ill and Defective in the United States. 1938. The National Committee for Mental Hygiene, New York. 151 pp.

NEW YORK
  New York City
    Bellevue Psychiatric Hospital and New York University
    New York State Psychiatric Institute and Hospital and Columbia
      University
  Thiells
    Letchworth Village

OHIO
  Columbus
    Columbus State Hospital and Ohio State University

WISCONSIN
  Madison
    Wisconsin Psychiatric Institute and University of Wisconsin

CHAPTER III
General Findings

IN general, this study of psychiatric research activities under private auspices follows the lines of the earlier study of research activities, facilities and potentialities in public institutions for the mentally ill and defective. Its purpose is essentially the same, namely, to present an informative picture of the status of psychiatric research in the United States, which may serve as a base line for future operations and measures looking toward the strengthening of scientific work in the field of mental and nervous diseases.

The present report, like the earlier one, is essentially descriptive and does not undertake a critical appraisal of research work. Nor does it attempt an evaluation and rating of clinical facilities, as was done in the first report, in terms of factor analysis, to determine the capacities of mental hospitals for investigative work. The situation in regard to private research centers is in many respects so unlike that of public institutions as to require a somewhat different type of approach and treatment and hence a different form of presentation.

In the first place, there are many more centers of research activity under private auspices, with a greater diversity in patterns of organization and function and more extensive community relationships than is the case with state hospitals. These differences are apparent from the descriptions of the research centers themselves and are further elaborated in other chapters of this report. In the second place, there is the prominent differentiating factor represented by the far greater number of medical schools and institutions associated with them that are involved in the present study. We are therefore dealing, to some extent, with a different set of facts and circumstances, and it is the character of the material deriving from them that shapes the character of the present report. While the

13

material does not lend itself to fine statistical analysis, a few pertinent facts and figures may be adduced. The larger findings and significances are interpreted in the chapter on "General Considerations and Conclusions." Here we summarize some of the more obvious findings.

Distribution of Research Facilities

To begin with, we find that, as in the earlier study, the larger concentration of psychiatric research activity is in the institutions in New England, along the Atlantic seaboard, and in the East North Central States. Only 7 of the 22 states represented in the group covered by this study are west of the Mississippi.

It is interesting to note that of the 100 facilities listed, only 25 are private mental hospitals, representing about 10 per cent of all private mental institutions in the country. The remainder are medical schools (26), general hospitals (21), clinics (6), public mental hospitals (4), and other institutions and agencies (18). No estimate is made of the extent of research activity in private mental hospitals as compared with other centers. As some of the most active research centers are included in this group of institutions, no inference is drawn except that there is a wider spread of psychiatric research interest and activity among centers other than private mental hospitals.

With the addition of the 10 medical schools associated with the research centers described in the first study, there are altogether 36, or more than half of all Class "A" medical schools in the country, that engage in psychiatric research.

Indicative of the extensive inter-relations of the various research centers with other centers in their respective communities and beyond, is the fact that over 170 institutions and agencies are named with which affiliations have been established, besides many others not identified by name.

Range of Research Interests

The descriptive reports on the research centers, given in Chapters V, VI, and VII, outline the general character of the researches they are respectively engaged in. These narratives are based largely on information obtained through personal visits to the various centers. Subsequently, those in charge of research activities were requested to furnish a list of research projects, by title, now in progress at their centers. In most of the responses to our request the researches under way were specified in more or less detail, while in others the projects were characterized in general terms, presumably to guard against premature disclosure of confidential aspects of the work. The subjects of study, as listed and defined in these replies, appear in Appendix "A".

Analysis of this supplementary information shows a distribution of research activity and interest of considerable range and scope. An attempt was made to classify the projects according to the classification employed by the Index Medicus. This could be done only approximately, as many of the projects cover two or more fields of study and fall into one category as readily as another. The tabulation below is therefore not a cumulative one, adding up to so many separate and distinct projects. Taking the studies by title, as listed in the returns from the various centers, there is an estimated total of 600 project entities, but many of these ramify and overlap into several categories of investigation. The following index is intended to show the distribution of studies in terms of these categories.

Clinical studies, it will be seen, lead the list, comprising numerically the largest single classification. Taken together with studies in therapy and those in clinical psychology and general medicine, they account for a majority of the projects. Indicative, however, of the broad scope of present day "psychiatric" research, and the growing interest in the constitutional and physical bases of mental and nervous disorders, are the impressive number of studies dealing with problems in organic neurology, neuroanatomy and neuropathology, neurophysiology, biochemistry and allied medical sciences. About 40 per cent of the projects fall into these fields, those under neurophysiology and biochemistry representing the most numerous single

Subject Classification	Number of Studies
Clinical, neurological and psychiatric *...............	227
Clinical, convulsive disorders.........................	21
Therapy (except those under next headings)..........	15
Shock therapy	33
Psychotherapy, including medical psychology.........	27
Biochemistry and clinical laboratory †................	90
Neuroanatomy and neuropathology...................	46
Neurophysiology and experimental psychology ‡.......	119
Constitutional, heredity, etc.........................	11
Endocrine and vegetative nervous system............	23
Growth studies	25
Administration and statistics........................	9
Psychiatric aspects of general medicine.............	55

* Including clinical psychology.
† Including pharmacological experiments.
‡ Including electroencephalography and general physiology.

classifications next to "clinical." Significant also of the "psychosomatic" trend is the substantial number of studies of the psychiatric aspects of general medicine. In all these respects, the distribution as to types of study in the present report differs markedly from that noted in the previous report. In the research centers under public auspices, the investigations described were predominantly of a therapeutic and clinical nature, while those on the physical and laboratory side were relatively few.

Personnel Engaged in Research

Information was also sought as to the professional personnel engaged in psychiatric research at the various centers. A list of the workers reported, with their names and the positions they hold, appears in Appendix "B". They include not only those who are responsible for directing or conducting the researches in progress, but also those who are participating in them in an important way. The list is probably not complete, as we have reason to believe that the reporting in some instances was limited to workers more closely identified with psychiatric departments and did not embrace those who are contributing to psychiatric research from other departments of scientific investigation. It is apparent, however, that non-psychiatric investigators in considerable numbers are collaborating in psychiatric research projects whose scope, as we have seen above, extends frequently to other fields of scientific study. A tally of the names reported shows an approximate numerical distribution, by professional categories, as follows:

Psychiatry and neuropsychiatry	275
Neurology	26
Psychology	55
General medicine	14
Pediatrics	12
Anatomy	8
Physiology	13
Pathology	8
Biophysics	6
Biochemistry and pharmacology	16
Surgery	4
Cardiology	3
Anesthesiology	2
Ophthalmology	1
Psychiatric social work	15
Applied sociology	1
Anthropology	2
Nursing	5
Occupational therapy	2
Education and physical education	8
Medical statistics	4
Unclassified	51
Total	531

Financing Research

An attempt was made to ascertain the extent and the sources of the financial support available for research work. This phase of our inquiry was only partially productive as we were faced with limitations inherent in the natural reticence of research establishments in reporting freely data of this character. Most of the centers indicated frankly enough the general sources of their research funds and many were quite specific, but only a few gave full information, with the result that nothing like definite figures are at hand from which to estimate the sum total of funds invested in psychiatric research under private auspices. Some centers reported lump sum appropriations covering salaries for teaching and clinical work as well as research, and for reasons of bookkeeping could not readily furnish differentiated figures. There was also the obvious difficulty of recording, to say nothing of measuring in terms of dollars and cents, the time devoted to research by individual investigators who pursue their studies without benefit of special funding.

Nevertheless, the information tendered by the various centers, and summarized in Appendix "C" of this report, has a certain value for the light it throws on the problem of securing adequate and sustained support for a hitherto neglected and, financially speaking, relatively undeveloped field of scientific activity. The reports show a "turn in the tide" and an increasing trend of support of psychiatric research on the part of Foundations and Funds and other benefactors. Many of these are named, others are referred to anonymously. The reports also show, on the other hand, the extent to which the slenderest resources have been taken advantage of and put to work for scientific ends wherever psychiatric research is favorably regarded and the slightest opportunities for original investigation present themselves. Often this scientific spirit is expressed under handicaps and accompanied by sacrifice, as in one center where fees for teaching are turned back into a common research fund, and in another center where consultation fees are pooled for research purposes. In others, research funds have been built up systematically through modest allotments from institutional income, from patients' fees, private earnings and other increments. Donations from grateful patients represent a promising source of support in some instances. In several places help has come from government sources, such as the Works Progress Administration and the National Youth Administration. More frequently research work has been made possible by the contributions of scientific staffs themselves and by the liberal policies of enlightened and progressive administrators who manage somehow to provide for it under their regular institutional budgets.

CHAPTER IV
Types of Research Center

The Rôle of the Private Institution

THE difference between the public and the private institution in the prosecution of research must be thought of as a trend of emphasis, which may or may not exist in actuality, but which is likely to exist. As a rule, the private institution is smaller and more responsive to the decisions of one person, is more limited in its clinical material, and is more subject to the necessity of being self-supporting, sometimes plus a margin of profit. Its research activities are apt to be less programmed, more restricted in number and variety, and more expressive of some individual interest. Still, every one of these characteristics may disappear in the individual case.

The proprietary hospital whose whole service is of the treatment type, whether of a high order or not, naturally did not enter seriously into this report. A few hospitals of lesser standing, clinically or otherwise, claimed to be doing research, but this claim was clearly unwarranted.

In evaluating research status, there are two rather important groups of private hospitals to be differentiated, namely, the proprietary and the voluntary.* The proprietary hospital, personally owned and operated by a person or group of persons, is more individualistic, whereas the voluntary hospital conducted by a board of trustees through employed staff, is more subject to group thinking. These, again, are not absolutely distinct, since some of the proprietary institutions have in whole or in part been made foundations, while some of the voluntary hospitals

---

* The term "voluntary" is used to denote the private, non-proprietary type of hospital; the term "proprietary" applies to private hospitals owned by persons or corporations and conducted for profit. Most large non-public general hospitals are voluntary institutions.

21

have become very much the expression of one person. In general, however, the research interest of one person in the proprietary hospital colors the research activity of that institution. This has distinct values, for it provides an intensity and a continuity of attention that are usually very productive. The Menninger Sanitarium, the Austen Fox Riggs Foundation, and Gladwyn Colony are good examples of this tendency. The voluntary hospital, on the other hand, has a variety of research interests more or less group-determined and continuous beyond the tenure of individuals. One identifies these institutions very seriously with research, but not so definitely with a particular research.

The Rôle of the Medical School

The consistency with which medical schools have pursued research reflects their special capacity to perform this function. Psychiatric problems, reflecting as they do every aspect of human behavior, have a special need for studies made with many kinds of laboratory and technical consultation aids. The selection of faculty personnel usually involves a consideration of the research contributions or potentialities of candidates, and so the stage is set for research more consistently in the medical school than at any other place. Psychiatry has not fared as well as other branches of medicine in this respect in the past, but new developments in the medical schools, such as the increase in provisions for psychiatric teaching and the organization of new psychiatric departments, are changing the picture for the better.

The Value of the Research Complex

Just as the proprietary and the voluntary hospitals have certain special values in the conduct of research that are distinct from each other and from those of the medical school, so there is a transcendent value in the integration of these values. The sum of the research facilities in certain communities is less than the research values of the complex of these centers. Usually this complex is the result of geographical proximity. Sometimes it derives from the continued cohesion of workers and students from a certain focus. The interlocking of staff appointments and the use of common facilities bridges the gaps between centers in the complex.

CHAPTER V

Reports of Medical School Centers

ALBANY, N. Y.

Albany Hospital and Albany Medical College

PSYCHIATRY in Albany, New York, centers in the departments of neurology and psychiatry of the Albany Hospital and the Albany Medical College, which share the same appointees as department heads. In both the hospital and the college there is a long-standing interest in psychiatry, the pioneer psychiatric unit of a general hospital having been established here.

These institutions are also an integral part of the community and have established intimate relations with various community agencies. The nursing school of the hospital is an affiliate of Russell Sage College, where preclinical nursing training is given. The department of psychiatry * gives abundant consultation to other departments and collaborates especially closely with the department of medicine. The department has no laboratories of its own, but there are research and clinical laboratories in which practically every need can be met. The physiological and pharmacological research laboratories are particularly productive in studies of brain metabolism. They are equipped with electroencephalographic apparatus, animal experimentation facilities, temperature regulation, and visual dark room. The department shares a central library which contains the important standard works and psychiatric periodicals.

The clinical facilities of this center include provision for 34 psychiatric and 10 neurological in-patients. Some 900 patients pass through this department each year. The

* We refer to ''the department'' in the singular since for practical purposes the psychiatric departments in the hospital and the college function as one.

out-patient service receives about 4,000 patient-visits a
year. There is a staff of 11 physicians and 13 nurses.
Cases of all types are admitted. The average stay of
patients is about two weeks, 30 days being the usual limit
for observation and temporary care and treatment pending commitment to other institutions.

The department has consultative connections with a
number of community institutions and agencies. The
Hudson Training School for Girls shares with the department a psychiatrist who conducts the Child Psychiatric
Out-patient Service at Albany. Consultative service is also
given the Berkshire Industrial School for Boys. These
boys are also served by the out-patient section. Similar
service is given weekly to the Protestant Family Welfare
Society, and the State Department of Health finances a
project of the department whereby neurosyphilitic patients
who have no behavior difficulties are given intensive anti-
syphilitic treatment. The Juvenile Court calls on the
department frequently for advice on its cases. On the
other hand, some of the social work of the hospital is conducted by community agencies.

There has been a continuous reporting of researches
from this center over a period of years. These researches
are of both the clinical and the laboratory types. The
close collaboration between the psychiatric department
and the department of physiology and pharmacology is
shown in the study of brain metabolism, especially with
reference to oxygen changes both in animals and in clinical
cases of psychoses. Experiments are directed toward the
alteration of symptoms by experimental oxygen changes
and, similarly, toward the modification of pathological
conditions. New approaches are being sought to the study
of memory. Experimentation is under way with erythroidin as a therapeutic agent. An effort is being made to
develop a ''case study'' of the community of Albany, in
terms of the human factors that enter into the growth and
development of that community.

AUGUSTA, GA.

University of Georgia School of Medicine and University Hospital

Psychiatric research at the University of Georgia is centered at the university hospital under the direction of the professor of psychiatry of the school of medicine. There are no psychiatric wards as such, all psychiatric patients being admitted to the general medical wards of the hospital, where little or no attempt is made to segregate them from other types of patient. In spite of this admittedly unsatisfactory arrangement, there is a workable and productive program of investigative activities, buttressed by an effective system of interdepartmental collaboration for research and teaching purposes, in which all the scientific workers are members of the faculty of the medical school and are on the staff of the university hospital. Those from the departments of psychiatry, medicine, anatomy, pathology and physiology are particularly active in their use of the available research facilities. A unique feature is the so-called four-year joint teaching plan for the nervous system adopted by the departments of anatomy, neuropsychiatry and neurosurgery.

The hospital has a fairly well equipped laboratory, with a pathologist and laboratory technicians, and autopsies are performed whenever possible. The library is quite modern, containing all the recent standard texts, practically all the medical journals, and seven neuropsychiatric journals. It is extensively used and the newer literature is freely discussed at staff conferences. The department of anatomy maintains a research laboratory exclusively devoted to problems of the nervous system and an exchange of men and materials is effected with the American Otological Society laboratory in the department of psychology at the University of Rochester, where neuro-electrical studies are carried out.

Special studies on the psychopathic personality were recently completed, and various current research projects have to do with malnutrition and with shock therapies in the psychoses. Special studies are in progress on prolonged non-hypoglycemic coma during insulin therapy. The department of neuropsychiatry is also working in conjunction with the department of internal medicine on the avitaminoses.

DETROIT, MICH.

Wayne University and Eloise Hospital

The connection between Wayne University and Eloise Hospital (a county mental hospital) is so close, in the fields both of psychiatry and of social service work, that the activities of the two institutions are inseparable at many points. Nearly all of the researches of the former are carried out at and financed through the latter. A few projects are undertaken, in addition, at Harper Hospital, a general voluntary hospital.

Eloise Hospital, one of the largest county institutions for mental diseases in the country, serves practically all the functions usually performed by a state hospital, its high per capita expenditure permitting it to do more than the average state hospital in many aspects of its work. It has a staff of 25 psychiatrists, including a director of psychiatric research, some 17 social workers besides five students in social work, and an extensive consulting staff which links it with practically all the Detroit hospitals. Also, several of its staff members hold teaching positions at Wayne University College of Medicine and the University of Michigan.

The institution accommodates some 3,800 patients. It has, in addition, a large parole clinic, with the unsual provision, both at the clinic and within the hospital, that as far as possible and feasible the patient retains the same psychiatrist throughout the course of his treatment. The library facilities of the hospital are not well organized, but all the important psychiatric publications and many other periodicals and standard works are available. Laboratory facilities exist beyond the current demand for research, which is chiefly clinical.

Eloise Hospital affiliates with Harper Hospital to provide psychiatric training for nurses, and several universities in other parts of the country send psychologists there for clinical training. These psychologists often engage in research along the lines of their own interests. Students in social work from Wayne University, who receive field training here, also pursue studies in fulfillment of their academic requirements. These students also receive formal instruction from the psychiatric staff.

Research by members of the hospital staff is very strongly encouraged as a part of their training, and special supervision is provided. There is a very distinct and continuing interest in research through hypnosis, many reports on which have already been published. In addition, special studies are carried on, as unusual clinical opportunities for these present themselves. Special attention is being devoted to a protracted study of post-hypnotic behavior. A case of dual personality is the subject of a long-time follow-up study. Symbolism of written language is a continuing interest.

Some studies of shock treatment are included in the program. The use of metrazol in various depressive states and sinusoidal (electric) shock in sub-convulsive doses are being experimented with. An effort is under way, through special tests, to clarify the psychologic performance and muscular-coördination characteristics of paretic patients that may have prognostic value, and similar indicators of the value of shock treatment are being studied. A study of tuberculous patients for the purpose of elucidating mental characteristics is under way. Also, aside from their work with psychotic cases, staff members examine many persons charged with homicide for the courts in the state.

The unusual parole facilities of the hospital motivate a special interest in experimentation in the community adjustment of patients. One staff member is especially assigned to the re-evaluation of patients in the wards for whom there is no active treatment program. These offer potential rather than realized research opportunities.

The research by Wayne University carried on at Harper Hospital is primarily electroencephalographic, but it includes also special projects growing out of provocative clinical cases.

MINNEAPOLIS—ST. PAUL, MINN.

University of Minnesota and Minnesota General Hospital

Practically all of the researches carried on in psychiatry in the Twin Cities center in the division of nervous and mental diseases of the department of medicine of the University of Minnesota Medical School. This department has close relationships and interlocking staff appointments with other departments of the university and with several community agencies.

The Minnesota General Hospital, which is the chief clinical resource of the medical school, has both in-patient and out-patient services in psychiatry and a unique department of child psychiatry which unites psychiatry and pediatrics. The in-patient service is a modern unit of 37 psychiatric and 20 neurologic beds, well staffed and equipped for special therapeutic work, and it is prepared to treat all types of psychiatric patient.

Many of the research activities of this center reflect the union of neurology and psychiatry, in one functional division, and numerous reports, primarily of a research character, have been issued along neurological, neuropathological, clinical and neuro-psychiatric lines. Some of these are based upon studies of animals for which there are special facilities. The presence of a psychological staff in this department and inter-staff appointments in the department of psychology and the testing bureau of the university account for the unique studies undertaken, wherein tests are being developed to reveal or to measure various behavior and personality manifestations. Masculinity and femininity, hypochondriasis, and aphasia have already been studied in this way. Another type of investigation centers on child psychiatry, with a special orientation toward psychiatric problems of particular interest to the pediatrician, especially those of enuresis. The research productivity of this center is evidenced by many publications.

A close working relationship between the medical school and the Minnesota General Hospital and Ancker Hospital (St. Paul) brings these hospitals into contact with the rich laboratory and personnel resources of the university and makes available to the medical school a wide range of clinical material. In addition to these local hospitals, the graduate school of the university has an affiliation with the Mayo Clinic. This likewise represents a rich potential resource for research, demanding the special personnel and the specialized laboratory facilities to be found only in that center.

As already indicated, there are close relationships between the psychiatric department and other departments of the medical school as well as other schools of the university. Some of these, such as those with the psychology department and the testing bureau, have already been productive. Internal medicine and pediatrics work closely with psychiatry, and there are well-worn pathways between psychiatry and the student health service, from which several psychiatric reports have emanated, and the department of education.

NASHVILLE, TENN.

Vanderbilt University School of Medicine

Psychiatric and related investigations in Nashville are largely due to the stimulation of Vanderbilt University Medical School. But this focus in the state capital depends upon and often expresses itself through the state departments of health and institutions.

The departments of psychiatry, pediatrics, and pharmacology in the medical school coöperate intimately in their service as well as in their investigatory work. The department of psychiatry is limited in its clinical resources. There are a few in-patient consultation cases, but its major clinical material is in an out-patient clinic. It has, however, a close working relationship with the nearby state hospital through which it carries on chemo-therapeutic experiments with products prepared by the pharmacological department.

The department of pediatrics is especially concerned with experimentation in pediatric training looking toward the assumption of greater responsibility by pediatricians for handling the behavior problems of their patients. In this it collaborates closely with the department of psychiatry.

The state department of health is conducting an epidemiological study of psychiatric and mental health problems in a nearby rural district, in Williamson County, to determine the incidence of various types of problems, with the aim of setting up corrective measures. While under the full authority and leadership of the health department, this project enjoys the support and has access to the resources of the medical school, which is also conducting an educational program for the regular staff of the Williamson County health department.

NEW YORK, N. Y.

The New York Hospital—Cornell University Medical College

Payne Whitney Psychiatric Clinic
The New York Hospital—Westchester Division, White Plains, N. Y.

Psychiatric research in this group is definitely centered in the *Payne Whitney Psychiatric Clinic,* which is the psychiatric clinical center of The New York Hospital and the psychiatric teaching center of Cornell University Medical College. Characteristic of this medical center is the leveling of all barriers between departments, whereby not only clinical service, but research and education become collaborative functions and reflect more fully the integrated approach to the patient as a whole. The department of medicine, for example, has joined with psychiatry in so many ways that functional collaboration between the two is very simple. The same is true of the relations between pediatrics and psychiatry. With public health, surgery, and other clinical departments the road to collaboration is clear although not so abundantly traveled as yet.

The Payne Whitney Clinic has an in-patient service for 89 adults, and an out-patient service with a special children's division. There is also a nursery school division for children without abnormalities. All of these services are available and used for research, both in the field of pathological manifestations and in that of behavior and personality deviations among the relatively normal. The clinic is well equipped with laboratories—eight of them for internal medicine and biochemical work and seven for neurological investigations. Both of these services are fully staffed. There is also a group of psychological laboratories which are adequately equipped for extensive and varied researches, but are not as yet completely staffed. The psychology department is at present carrying out limited investigative work.

Very significant is the fact that the men in charge of these laboratories have appointments not only in the department of psychiatry, but also in the respective departments of medicine in the hospital or in the medical school. Researches emanating from the laboratories, and from the joint efforts of clinical workers in psychiatry, medicine, pediatrics, etc., are subsequently subjected to critical review by the two or more departments under which they are conducted. This is stimulating to the research and teaching activities of the collaborating departments, as well as scientifically broadening, in that these collaborative researches are often followed by individual related projects set up within the separate departments. In addition to this collaboration between clinical departments, joint researches are carried on with the basic science departments of anatomy, physiology and pharmacology.

There are facilities for animal experimentation not only within the psychiatric department, but in other departments as well, and these are mutually available as needed. Electroencephalo- and myographic apparatus are jointly used.

In addition to these clinical and laboratory facilities there are abundant library resources. The psychiatric library contains the important foreign and domestic psychiatric periodicals and the time-tested as well as the more recent monographs, reports and other books. There is also an unusual collection of older works, chiefly of historical value. A psychiatric history of the New York Hospital is now in preparation. An important aspect of the library is the functional cataloguing of the periodical literature whereby the literature on any psychiatric topic is easily located. A similar cataloguing of the records of clinical cases greatly facilitates their use for research purposes. In addition to this special library, the main library of the medical center is available nearby.

Besides the departmental relationships that are of value to research within this center, there are those that have been established with independent community agencies. These will become apparent in connection with certain collaborative projects referred to below.

It is difficult to classify the various threads of interest that run through successive research projects because of the multi-dimensional nature of these interests, and an attempt merely to list them would necessitate much duplication. It may be pointed out, however, that there is a tendency to direct a major part of the research activity toward the understanding of human psychology, or lesser psychopathology, as contrasted with that of the psychoses. Studies of emotions, for example, especially studies of fear and tension, involve contributory researches by several departments, such as metabolic, biochemical, neurological and neurophysiological investigations.

One group of studies is pointed toward the evaluation of cultural factors; late-life psychoses not obviously organic in origin involve these as well as psychopathological factors. A study of socio-economic factors in well-to-do patients has raised the issue of the application of social service to this class. The function of religion as a factor in adjustment is given special attention and study. The bearing of cultural factors on the management of sickness is the subject of another study facilitated by a coöperative relationship with the Community Service Society, a large private family case work agency; and this, in turn, has led to a study of the rôle of the psychiatrist in a family agency.

Another group of studies has to do with the genetics of personality. Specific facets of these studies include speech deviations, enuresis, anxiety and fear in children. The nursery school, which cares for 18 children and has a full-time teacher, is used for checking purposes in these studies. Special attention is paid to the psychology and the psychopathology of eating habits. Not limited to children is a study of confusion in thinking and of retention disorders.

Psychosomatic studies are directed to endocrine factors, with special reference to cyclic changes in young persons. In collaboration with pediatrics a study is being made of sweating in emotional states. Peptic ulcers are investigated psychobiologically, and electroencephalographic studies are made of confusion states. In this phase of research close contact is maintained with experiments in electroencephalography in other places. Electromyographic studies of tension states are in progress. These psychosomatic studies call for frequent joint undertakings with various departments. A clinical study of leucocytosis involves psychiatry, biochemistry and physiology. A study of loss of weight involves psychiatry, metabolism, animal experimentation, endocrinology and anatomy, as do studies of over-activity and anorexia nervosa. A special effort is being made to incorporate psychiatric elements into medical history taking and to train pediatricians and psychiatrists in the simpler procedures of psychological testing. On the therapeutic side, studies of the use of hypothermia involve laboratory and clinical assistance from several departments.

The *Westchester Division of the New York Hospital* has been a leading psychiatric center for many decades, contributing richly to the scientific literature and to clinical standards. It is a voluntary hospital administered as a separate institutional unit under the Society of the New York Hospital. It is located at White Plains, convenient to New York City.

The hospital provides for approximately 350 male and female patients and has some 15 psychiatrists on its staff. Its clinical resources are of a high order, as attested by its long-standing leadership in the field of occupational therapy and its traditional ideals of care and treatment of the mentally ill. The adjunct facilities of the hospitals include a professional library of some 5,000 standard volumes and the important psychiatric periodical literature. Weekly staff conferences are held for review and discussion of the literature or special scientific topics and for the presentation of scientific reports.

The clinical laboratory, which regularly employs two technicians and is in charge of one staff psychiatrist, is well suited for research studies, its actual use depending upon investigations in progress. It is equipped with electroencephalograph, inductotherm, electric shock and other diagnostic and therapeutic apparatus. Research by the staff is a part of the hospital policy and assistance is provided for this purpose, but the researches themselves tend to follow the individual interests of staff members. From time to time patients are especially admitted in order to facilitate certain research studies. There are autopsy facilities and a high autopsy rate. Neuropathological work is conducted at the New York Hospital in New York City. The staff of the Westchester Division is closely affiliated with the New York Hospital and Cornell University Medical School, where the medical director is professor of clinical psychiatry and three other staff members have teaching and out-patient clinical appointments. There, also, a New York City office of the Westchester Division is maintained for contacts with or about former, current, or prospective patients. Two other staff members attend this service. Others have, at times, appointments to Vanderbilt Clinic and the Neurological Institute—both affiiliated with Columbia University and with the Dental School of New York University. Under an arrangement of considerable practical value with the New York State Psychiatric Institute at the Columbia Medical Center, a staff member may be released from his clinical duties at the Westchester Division, although retained on the staff, in order to take three months' training in neuropathology at the Institute. In addition, the hospital has teaching affiliations for student nurses from the following hospitals: Mt. Sinai, Flower-Fifth Avenue, Presbyterian, Roosevelt, St. Luke's, Mt. Vernon, White Plains, Syracuse General, and Methodist Episcopal of Brooklyn.

The research activities of the hospital are, in general, inclined toward the clinical. They include adaptations and evaluations of the shock therapies, with chemical, psychological and hematological studies of patients, and prognosticating factors. Convulsions following withdrawal of sedatives are of special interest. Clinical features of arteriosclerotic psychoses are being analyzed. There are also studies of the psychopathic personality, the therapy of alcoholic patients, and a long-term study of psychoneurotic patients. Psychosomatic studies, clinical and biochemical studies of sex function and dysfunction, electrocardiographic studies, and studies of heredity reflect other research interests.

New York Post Graduate Hospital and Medical School

This institution is affiliated with Columbia University, but functionally it is practically autonomous, owing in part to the distance from the Columbia Medical Center.* It provides hospital facilities in many specialties, although there are no in-patient psychiatric facilities. Psychiatry is practiced chiefly through an out-patient clinic and through consultations on in-patients. The institution also provides regular post-graduate courses and clinical conferences. The medical staff is psychoanalytically oriented and has the adjunct services of a sociologist and a psychologist. There are 11 psychiatrists and 35 neurologists. There is a small working library, which includes the standard psychiatric journals, but for more detailed studies the libraries of Columbia University are used.

Psychiatric research is primarily clinical and, while individually oriented, tends to follow two lines. Several studies, already reported, are in the field of intra-family relations, with special reference to psychopathological factors in emotional divorce. Other studies are pointed toward the analysis of behavior problems of children, in which there is joint interest with the department of pediatrics. In the prosecution of both sets of studies the department of psychiatry has available to it the laboratory and consultation facilities of the hospital for routine tests and analyses and for roentgenological work.

OMAHA, NEB.

University of Nebraska Medical School

> *Bishop Clarkson Memorial Hospital*
> *Douglas County Hospital*

While research efforts in Omaha are primarily dependent on individual initiative, those engaged in psychiatric investigation are associated with the University of Nebraska Medical School, whose clinical and laboratory resources

* The facilities for psychiatric research at the Columbia Medical Center are centered at the New York State Psychiatric Institute and Hospital and have been previously reported. (See *Research in Mental Hospitals:* A Survey and Tentative Appraisal of Research Activities, Facilities and Possibilities in State Hospitals and Other Tax-Supported Institutions for the Mentally Ill and Defective in the United States. New York. 1938. The National Committee for Mental Hygiene. 151 p.)

are available. Omaha is unusually well equipped with psychiatric resources in its general hospitals. The *Bishop Clarkson Memorial Hospital* is especially active as a research center. It has a small neuro-psychiatric department of 30 beds and is well equipped with modern therapeutic adjuncts. All types of patient can be treated without restraint. Affiliate psychiatric nursing courses are given. The psychiatric residency and nursing departments are accredited.

The psychiatric facilities in conjunction with the medical school have been continually productive in research and numerous reports have been issued. The studies are clinical in nature and deal especially with chemotherapeutic agents, their effects, and their adaptation to various psychoses. Pioneer work on convulsive shock therapy in affective disorders was begun here. Distinctive work has been done on the use of curare in preventing complications in shock treatment. Special attention has also been given to the application of induced fever to the treatment of infectious diseases, especially those of the central nervous system. A special Fever Therapy Research department has been organized and collaborates with the state hospital service.

Closely related to the department of neuro-psychiatry of the medical school also is the *Douglas County Hospital,* with which staff appointments are exchanged. The psychiatric department of this hospital has an average population of 165 patients, and an average monthly admission rate of 35 new patients. These patients are largely psychotic, the remainder being alcoholic and drug addiction patients. Insulin therapy was first introduced in this hospital in 1936, and in connection with the psychiatric department of the Methodist Hospital, bio-chemical and clinical studies of insulin have been made and were reported in 1937. Reports on metrazol therapy in the depressions, as carried out in this hospital and in the Methodist and Lutheran Hospitals, have also been made. During the past year, in conjunction with the Lutheran Hospital, a study of the intravenous use of magnesium sulphate, to prevent excessive muscular contraction and bone fractures in metrazol and electric shock therapy, has been carried out.

PORTLAND, ORE.

University of Oregon Medical School

Investigations at the University of Oregon Medical School are of a clinical type. The department of psychiatry, working closely with medicine and surgery, has centered its attention on therapeutic work with psychoneurosis, especially on a short-term and rational basis, such as may be carried over into general practice. It is also experimenting with the application of child psychiatry under the limiting conditions of a rural setting on a state-wide basis.

The department consists of seven psychiatrists, most of them in private practice in Portland. Cases from private practice as well as those from the out-patient psychiatric and the medical and surgical services are all considered a research resource of the department.

Members of the department act as directive and administrative heads for a state-wide traveling child guidance clinic whose cases are likewise available for research. Recent additions provide neuro-pathological laboratory and encephalographic facilities.

The high suicide rate in the locality has attracted the attention of the department toward investigation of this problem. A project for aiding physicians of the state in the handling of psychoneuroses is being investigated with the coöperation of the State Board of Health.

SYRACUSE, N. Y.

Syracuse Psychopathic Hospital and Syracuse University

All of the psychiatric research interests of Syracuse University center at the Syracuse Psychopathic Hospital which, while it is a New York State institution operating under the Department of Mental Hygiene, functions as the psychiatric department of the university. In addition to the research activities pursued by its own personnel, it offers opportunity to others in the university and in various institutions and agencies in the city to conduct research under its aegis. The hospital provides for 60 in-patients and has a well organized out-patient department for adults and children. Its services are mainly for individuals suffering from incipient mental disorders, including psychoneuroses, emotional and social maladjustments and behavior disorders of children, though it also receives definitely psychotic patients for observation and temporary treatment. It has an adequate full-time staff and good laboratory and library facilities. Its teaching and research relations with Syracuse University, while centered at the medical school, extend to other departments as well, and collaborative researches have been and are carried on with several of them, as also with the State Department of Education. It also receives students from the New York School of Social Work whose training includes a research dissertation.

While there is a general research interest among all members of the hospital's staff, three of them are especially inclined toward investigative work. Many researches have been carried out in this center and the literature contains many evidences of its scientific productiveness. Its research interests run heavily to children's problems, wherein special attention is given to the investigation of treatment techniques, educational disabilities, the experimental use of diagnostic tests, the diagnosis and classification of delinquencies, and the problems of institutional children.

On the adult side, the studies deal with involutional melancholia and alcoholic psychoses, with special reference to pre-psychotic manifestations, suicide, encephalitis, epilepsy, traumatic psychoses, especially those associated with head injuries, neuroses, somatic disorders, and the reactions to cryptorchidism. Continuous attention has been given to the clinical application of benzedrine and barbiturates in several neurological and psychiatric states.

CHAPTER VI

Reports of Research Complexes

BALTIMORE, MD.

Johns Hopkins University

> *Henry Phipps Psychiatric Clinic*
> *Harriet Lane Home*
> *School of Hygiene and Public Health*

WHILE the *Henry Phipps Psychiatric Clinic* is the functional center of psychiatric research in the complex of medical activities in Baltimore, its clinical and educational services throughout Johns Hopkins Hospital and the community provide a web of facilities that support much broader research activities and potentialities. The Harriet Lane Home, adjacent to Phipps Clinic, the School of Hygiene and Public Health, also close by, the neurological department and the endocrine division of internal medicine, all have formal research connections, while consultation service provided to the other departments of the hospital are closely related to a special psychosomatic program existing in its own right. In the community the out-patient department facilitates close relations with the schools and the social agencies. Regular psychiatric concultation service is provided to the juvenile court, supplementing the court's own regular psychiatrist, and one member of the Phipps' staff serves as psychiatrist to Goucher College. A formal arrangement exists between the Phipps Clinic and the state hospitals at Springfield and Spring Grove, whereby the facilities of both are united for professional education and research.

The Phipps Clinic houses the department of psychiatry of the *Johns Hopkins Medical School*. It has an in-patient service of some 80 beds, with facilities for patients of all clinical and economic classes. It has an out-patient department for children and adults. It is adequately staffed, for clinical purposes, with residents and fellows. The clinic has been widely recognized for its educational, clinical, and research leadership. It has clinical, psychobiological, neurological, reflex conditioning and animal laboratories. Practically all its staff physicians are active in some phase of research and reports are presented from time to time at staff conferences. Some 55 reports of studies by members of the Phipps' staff were published during 1940–1941.

The psychobiological laboratory has large quarters and equipment and both research and auxiliary staff for animal experimentation. It is carrying on extensive studies on reactions to alcohol and variations in Vitamin B. These studies involve broader investigations of taste and appetite and the influence of induced neurological and endocrine disturbances.

The clinical laboratory is set up for the necessary chemical studies of patients, but also has centered attention on a critical study of electrical shock treatment. Blood changes accompanying this form of treatment are being studied. The laboratory collaborates with the internal medicine department of the hospital on endocrinological studies conducted by the latter. It provides the electroencephalographic observations in Addison's disease and induced changes in potassium-sodium balance. These are of special interest because of the relationships of their symptomatology to that of neurasthenia. Electroencephalographic studies are also being made, in collaboration with the out-patient department, on a group of school children, in order to establish electroencephalographic norms checked with intelligence tests, teachers' reports and parents' interviews.

The Pavlovian Laboratory is studying differential conditioning, the production of experimental "neuroses" and the elimination of "neurosis" in animals, and the differences in conditioning of patients with different forms of psychosis. Korsakow's syndrome has been given special attention. The neurological laboratory is studying the neuropathological manifestations of animals subjected to metrazol, and the thalamic changes in sheep subjected to operative trauma.

On the clinical side, a survey and review is being made of all previous patients of the hospital. Out of this project specific studies have emerged, such as determination of the status of schizophrenic patients after some 25 years; an analysis of factors in patients in various classifications, especially the affective and psychoneurotic cases, looking toward a critical discussion of prognosis; and an analysis of recent cases for leads that may suggest further investigations. A critical study is being made of the results of shock therapy. The out-patient department is conducting, in one public school, a study of retarded children and delinquents and other behavior problems, and in another, a study of reading difficulties.

The house staff at this center provides consultation service to other departments of the hospital which have no special consulting psychiatrist and through this there is research collaboration. This includes studies of hypoglycemia in tension states, and psychiatric factors in internal medical problems, such as obesity and hypertension. The central files of the hospital include a statistical punch card system in which the psychiatric cases are classified and made easily available for special studies. The psychoneuroses, especially from other departments of the hospital, are recorded in considerable detail. The division of neurology collaborates very closely with the department of psychiatry.

The *Harriet Lane Home for Invalid Children* has its own psychiatric staff, who hold appointments with the department of psychiatry. They deal mostly with out-patients, but also provide consultation on in-patients. A long-time project of this staff is a follow-up study of 700 children over a period of years, undertaken as a test of the clinical effort. Experimental work is done in the teaching of psychiatry in pediatrics. The play interview, as a diagnostic and therapeutic approach to the child, is the subject of special study, and an analysis is being made of the awareness and the attitudes of children. Special attention is given to the problems of the mother who is shifting from an outside career to domestic life. Advantage is taken of opportunities to study isolated clinical problems offered by the occasional case, such as catalepsy, tics, age-problem relations. One member of the staff gives special attention to the resistance of children and its management and the affective display of children in relation to special persons and objects.

Likewise related, by joint participation, is the mental hygiene program of the *School of Hygiene and Public Health*. This includes a long-time study of a health district of Baltimore which is the urban phase of, and is related informally to, a rural study being carried out under other auspices in Franklin, Tennessee. This health district study includes a thorough canvass to elicit all mental hygiene cases. It is part of a general bio-statistical analysis of this district.

The Phipps' staff gives free psychiatric consulting service to the doctors of this district and to the various agencies in relation to pre-school children. It is attempting to work out techniques whereby mental hygiene can be applied prophylactically in this district through its existing resources.

Another phase of the mental hygiene problem is being studied jointly by the departments of medicine and of preventive medicine. The study consists of an investigation of the environmental and social problems presented by patients who are attending the general medical dispensary. Emphasis is being given in this study, and in teaching, to the total individual; and the conflicts, tensions and social problems of selected patients as factors in their illness are investigated and discussed in weekly conferences. This study serves to bring out not only the mental and personality disturbances that may accompany disease, but also the early manifestations of the neuroses and their causes, at a stage when simple methods of treatment may be effective.

BOSTON, MASS.

Harvard Medical School
Massachusetts General Hospital
McLean Hospital
Peter Bent Brigham Hospital
Boston City Hospital
Children's Hospital
Tufts College Medical School
Habit Clinic for Child Guidance
Beth Israel Hospital
Judge Baker Guidance Center

The *Massachusetts General Hospital* has a long record of contributions to medical research and, particularly during the past seven years, has steadily produced reports of psychiatric research. The hospital has special provision for some 18 mental patients, who are primarily psychoneurotics of the anxious and compulsive type, although it can also deal with the more disturbed. Moreover, the psychiatric department has an abundant consultation service for the rest of the hospital, whereby its own clinical resources are greatly amplified. Probably 500 patients a year are seen in this way, both for consultation and for continuous advice and collaborative treatment. Some of these patients may be transferred to the psychiatric department, while others come from the emergency ward and the out-patient service. The latter likewise receives most of its patients by reference from other departments. For studies of vegetative neurology many sympathectomized patients are available.

The department has a permanent staff of four full-time psychiatrists, one of whom directs the in-patient facility and research activities, and another the out-patient service. There are two resident psychiatrists, a psychologist, three social workers, and five social work students from Simmons and Smith Colleges. These students are chiefly in the out-patient service. There are one or two Rockefeller fellows and in the out-patient service a number of part-time psychiatrists.

The hospital has many local ties. Its staff members are all on the faculty of *Harvard Medical School*. Its work in neuropathology is coördinated in the same department with neurology and with the Boston Psychopathic Hospital. It shares the services of the psychologist of the Harvard Fatigue Laboratory. McLean Hospital for the mentally ill is coördinated with the Massachusetts General under the same board. They are functionally related also in that psychiatrists from McLean attend the Massachusetts General's out-patient department, and the staffs of the two institutions function in a mutual advisory capacity, with exchanges of personnel at staff meetings of both. At times studies at Massachusetts General include McLean patients. Students from the psychology department of the Harvard School of Public Health are used in connection with researches, and the head nurse of this department teaches in the Massachusetts General School of Nursing. More casual than continuous are the relationships with Boston State Hospital and Boston City Hospital.

The laboratory facilities of the psychiatric department are varied and, in general, well equipped. There are special resources for neuropathology, for electroencephalography, for studies on respiration, used especially in work on brain metabolism, and for Pavlovian conditioning, plithysmographic and skin resistance determinations, in addition to the various accessory facilities required for clinical work.

The psychiatric library resources are largely personal property, but the Boston Psychopathic and Boston Medical libraries are both readily accessible.

The research interests of this center are directed particularly toward the understanding and treatment of the psychoneurotic. These interests are in part clinical and in part concerned with more fundamental studies at the physiological level. The anxiety states and psychosomatic difficulties are especially considered and of the latter, dermatitis, asthma, arthritis, thyroid and post-operative states receive close attention.

Current researches include investigation both of basal functions and of response to unusual conditions. These investigations involve encephalographic, cardio-vascular, respiratory, conditioned reflex (salivary), and pain threshold studies, and the tendency is to use a multiple approach to a given problem. Even on the clinical side this multiple approach is expressed by joint clinical service by several departments, and instruction is offered to medical students in which the same cases are presented by different specialists. Biochemical studies accompany the physiological studies—for example, observations of P.H. in hyperventilation in neuroses. Interviewing involves studies of patients by more exact means, as for example with speech and visual records. Encephalograms and psychological tests are also employed to study levels of consciousness as affected by nitrous oxide.

Special attention is given to toxic cases, to post-operative effects (especially after hysterectomy), to Raynaud's disease in relation to neuroses, and to the use of red dyes as anti-convulsants. Electromyograms are used to reflect tensions, as in handwriting and tremor. Thyroid disorders are the subject of joint study with other departments.

McLean Hospital is a voluntary hospital for the mentally ill affiliated with the Massachusetts General Hospital, both institutions being under the same board. It has for many years been a center of intense research activity, and notable contributions have come continuously from its staff. Like the Massachusetts General Hospital, it has had close ties with Harvard University. It collaborates intimately with the Fatigue Laboratory of the Harvard School of Business Administration. Teaching is carried on at the medical school. There is collaboration at the Harvard Hygiene Clinic in a study of factors in the illness of college men and in a control study of "normal" students, and students with psychiatric problems that require hospital treatment are admitted here. Some members of McLean's staff give part-time service to the Massachusetts General out-patient department, and there is an exchange in attendance at staff meetings and consultations. The research program is under the advisement of leaders from the Boston Psychopathic and Boston State Hospitals. The hospital has its own nursing school, for both men and women, affiliating for its own students with Boston Lying-in Hospital, Children's Hospital, and Massachusetts General Hospital, and offering psychiatric training for students of Massachusetts General and Peter Bent Brigham Hospitals. It also assists Simmons College in the training of public health nurses.

The hospital has a rated capacity of 220 patients of all types, about 50 per cent of whom are from the metropolitan area, and there is a staff of 14 psychiatrists. The hospital has its own library, containing most of the current psychiatric periodicals, and it makes use of the Boston Medical and other libraries to supplement this. Its laboratories are well equipped for biochemical studies and it has a full-time biochemist on the staff. Its interest is directed toward brain tissue metabolism and vitamins. It has also a psychological laboratory with electroencephalographic equipment.

The researches of the hospital are primarily clinical. Various psychiatric approaches are provided for in its essentially psychobiological viewpoint. It gives special attention to physiological investigations. On the clinical side, it is studying the genetic background of manic-depressive states and has a full-time worker on this study. Another investigator is concentrating on case studies of suicidal symptoms, the rest of the staff collaborating. Special attention is given to experimentation in treatment. Insulin, metrazol and faradic treatments are being studied over a long period to determine their effects and by-effects. An attempt is under way to bring the faradic dosage under better control. Unique is the experimental use of hypo-thermia carried on in coöperation with the Fatigue Laboratory (which provides equipment) and with Massachusetts General Hospital (which provides internal medical and cardio-vascular supervision). The biochemical laboratory makes concurrent serological studies. Physiological studies accompanying recovery are designed to reflect pertinent changes. Another study of serological peculiarities of manic patients uses hypophis-ectomized and adrenal-ectomized cases as indicators.

The *Peter Bent Brigham Hospital* is a general hospital of 250 beds which provides medical and surgical service to adult patients. It has no special beds for neurological or psychiatric patients. It has, however, for years called regularly for psychiatric consultations in both its in-patient and out-patient services, and its internes, until recently, received part of their training at the Worcester State Hospital.

The hospital has a close relationship with Harvard Medical School, where its department heads hold professorial rank. It uses the Harvard and Boston Medical libraries and those of associated hospitals. There are overlapping appointments with the staff of Boston Psychopathic Hospital, which also collaborates on electroencephalographic studies, and of Boston City Hospital. The hospital has its own clinical laboratory facilities, but depends also, for special purposes, upon those of other hospitals nearby.

Of recent years the hospital staff has included a full-time psychiatrist, in addition to part-time psychiatrists, with a view to enriching the teaching of medical students and younger staff members. This psychiatrist holds hospital and medical school appointments in medicine. The psychiatric staff assists likewise in the education of nurses. The attempt is made, through the psychiatric staff, to develop methods of study appropriate to the non-psychotic patient that will produce pertinent personal and situational data bearing on his diagnosis and treatment. To this end the psychiatrists carry a regular medical function besides the purely psychiatric.

An out-patient psychiatric clinic facilitates the follow-up of special cases. One research study is directed toward an understanding of how patients feel about ward rounds for teaching purposes and how they behave in reaction to these. Another is an investigation of delirium as to its intellectual, emotional and physiologic aspects. There are occasional special follow-up studies of patients committed from the hospital. Investigation is also directed towards various neurophysiologic and neurologic phenomena.

Boston City Hospital is a public general hospital of 2,300 beds, with all the special services excepting the psychiatric. It has, however, a well equipped 60-bed neurological service for men, women and children. With these facilities, it can handle minor psychiatric disturbances, psychotic cases being evacuated promptly to state mental hospitals. Alcoholic patients are cared for on the medical wards. For its neurological (and psychiatric) needs, it has six internes and four residents. The residents give consultation service to other departments, arranging transfers when indicated, and they assist in neurosurgery. There are 17 visiting physicians in this service. There is an out-patient service three mornings a week, with 3,500 visits per year. Two afternoon clinics give special treatment for neurosyphilis and epilepsy, migraine and Parkinsonism, respectively, and the former also gives diagnostic service to rule out neurosyphilis.

The hospital, with its large staff, has many ties in the metropolitan area. Monson, Boston and Metropolitan state hospitals are especially close, the first through a common interest in epilepsy, the second through overlapping staff appointments, the third through mutual studies of neuropathological material. Numerous members of the Harvard University faculty are on the hospital staff. Tufts College and Boston University are also represented. Students from all three come for instruction. The hospital has its own nursing school. Its staff participates in the state neuropsychiatric course given at Metropolitan State

Hospital. Staff consultants serve also the Boston Dispensary, Peter Bent Brigham Hospital, and Cambridge City Hospital. Students of social work from Simmons College receive field training and lectures here, the department having two social workers on its staff, one for in-patient and one for out-patient service.

The laboratory facilities of the department are extensive and are devoted both to research and to clinical work. There are resources for animal experimentation, photography, electroencephalography, polarographic studies and blood chemistry. The department has a spinal fluid laboratory for the whole hospital. Three to five research fellows are occupied with experimental work.

The library facilities of the hospital include a central library and a smaller departmental library. It is not well equipped with psychiatric matter, but has a few periodicals. Chief dependence is placed on the Boston Medical Library.

There is abundant evidence in the literature of the research productivity of this center. It is the outstanding contributor to the study of epilepsy in this country. Its studies range over the clinical, sociological, therapeutic and electroencephalographic aspects of this disorder. A large corps of assistants is engaged in the electrical analysis of electroencephalographic records for various frequencies, and in attempts to determine the relationship of dysrhythmia to convulsive disorders, to other behavior manifestations, to heredity, to age, to migraine, and to schizophrenia. The circulation and the metabolism of the brain and the relation of these to dysrhythmia are also major subjects of inquiry. A search is under way for effective anti-convulsive drugs that are of therapeutic value, and for the chemical structure accountable for their efficacy. This effort extends to the treatment of rigidity and other disorders of movement. The epilepsy research, which requires about $25,000 annually, is financed for the most part by special grants from various foundations, by a pharmaceutical firm and by popular subscriptions made to the Harvard Epilepsy Commission.

A study of electrical activity of the brain is designed to clarify the relationship of cortex to basal ganglia and the effects of drugs applied to the cortex. Other related investigations deal with the sympathetic nervous system.

Various neuropathological studies deal with vitamin deficiencies, experimental injury, and the effects of disease processes. Attempts are also in progress to refine diagnostic and treatment procedures on patients with acute head and spinal injuries. Alcoholism is receiving considerable attention, including the development of therapy, analysis of factors, and other aspects of the disorder.

Ward 9 of the *Children's Hospital* has long been a link between pediatrics and psychiatry. The hospital is one of a group comprising the Harvard Medical School center. Into this ward of 14 beds come neurological and potentially neurological cases from the hospital, and children who need special observation and study find here special personnel, special play materials, quarters, and other requisite facilities. Assisting the psychiatrically oriented pediatrician who directs this department are a full-time psychologist, a play supervisor, nurses, nursing students and affiliates, a pediatric interne on a two-months' rotating service, and a social worker for follow-up and out-patient assistance. Consultation is exchanged with other departments of the hospital and out-patient service.

The Children's Hospital is closely related to Harvard Medical School through teaching appointments and classes for students conducted here, and there is provision for psychological internes. Lectures are also given to Simmons College students. The Judge Baker Guidance Center, the Boston Psychopathic Hospital, and local child-caring agencies all collaborate on the hospital's cases from time to time, and there are working relationships with other psychological and school services of the city. The hospital also maintains a convalescent home. The library facilities of the hospital, mainly general medical and pediatric, are supplemented by those of nearby Harvard

Medical School and Boston Psychopathic Hospital. The laboratories of the hospital serve Ward 9 as clinical adjuncts.

The research at this center is primarily clinical in nature, growing out of services to individual cases. In general, the emphasis in investigation is on the effects of structural disease upon growth and development. It is pointed toward the understanding of encephalopathic changes, their associated behavior changes, and the relation of these to situational influences on behavior. Experimental treatment procedures are related to these variables. Trauma, infections and diffuse (toxic) changes afford the major opportunity for investigation. Encephalographic facilities exist on the ward and are used for studies paralleling the clinical researches. Special attention is directed to cases of lead poisoning in relation to resultant obscure encephalopathies. The research also includes studies of delayed speech and the development of tests to reflect this delay.

While *Tufts College* faculty members are identified with psychiatric research activities under several other auspices, these are not primarily projects of the medical school, whose most intimate tie, through its professor of psychiatry, is with the *Habit Clinic for Child Guidance.*

The Habit Clinic was among the earliest of child guidance facilities in the country and a pioneer in such service for the younger child. It is a voluntary agency with many connections throughout Boston, and it provides clinical service to many of the welfare and health agencies of the community. Through its board membership, it has a tie with the Children's Hospital. It has a twenty-years' accumulation of case records, and its case experiences have been a major source of reference for the Federal Children's Bureau's publications on child development. The clinic serves children under ten years of age and receives about 200 cases per year. It has a staff of three part-time psychiatrists, a psychologist, two psychiatric social workers, and a pediatrician. One staff member devotes more than half-time to research.

The researches of the Habit Clinic are an outgrowth of its clinical work. It has long been interested in convulsive disorders and gives particular attention to the relation of infantile to later convulsions, and to mental deficiency and retardation. It has assisted in the study of children for purposes of adoption and has attempted to develop criteria of child and adoptive family characteristics that enhance the success of child placement. It is concerned also with the study of conduct disorders in relation to physical defects in children. The facilities of the Children's Hospital provide opportunities for observational studies of some children, and those of Beth Israel Hospital are especially called on for cases of eneuresis. The clinic is used as a field training center for students of social work from Simmons and Boston Colleges, and theses prepared by these students are often based on case material found here.

Beth Israel Hospital is a recently constructed general hospital of some 220 beds. There is no specific in-patient psychiatric service, but there is a psychiatric out-patient clinic. The hospital is chiefly related to Harvard University and is in close proximity to the medical school. Harvard carries a financial responsibility for several staff members. There are, however, also connections with Tufts College Medical School, and overlapping appointments with Boston State Hospital and other local and state institutions.

Owing to the nature of this hospital, its pertinent research contributions have been primarily in psychosomatic medicine, with special psychoanalytic perspective. It goes further, however, than the ordinary psychosomatic program, giving attention to the psychological concomitants and complications of physical disease. In this it is almost unique. On its staff are several psychiatrists who have contributed extensively to psychiatry. The present investigations in relation to problems of internal medicine have the sympathetic coöperation of the several depart-

ments of the hospital and the benefit of various technical
facilities. Special attention has been given to the study of
anorexia nervosa. The hospital has its own school of nursing. The character of its research interest also requires
special social service and psychiatric residents, provision
for which was recently made.

The *Judge Baker Guidance Center* has had an unbroken
record of some 25 years of scientific contributions to the
understanding of problems of conduct, personality and
education. It is a voluntary organization providing non-
residential psychiatric service to children. It serves chiefly
the Boston metropolitan area. Besides the two directors,
it has a clinical staff of three psychiatrists, one psycho-
therapist, two psychologists, and four social workers, some
of whom are qualified by training and experience for
psychoanalytic work. In addition, there are usually one
or two psychiatric fellowship holders, one psychological
assistant, and seven student psychiatric social workers. It
has a case record file dating back to 1917. Its cases are
regularly recorded by the Findex System, their research
value being thereby facilitated.

The center has extensive formal and informal connections with almost every functionally related institution in its
community. It has a long-established special coöperative
relationship with the juvenile courts of the vicinity. It
participates in the Citizenship Training School of the Boston Juvenile Court. It assists similarly, and receives cases
from, many community agencies and educational institutions for children. It uses the observational resources of
the Children's Hospital and the New England Home for
Little Wanderers.

The center accepts students for training from the schools
of social work of Boston University, Simmons College,
Boston College and Smith College, and assists these students in carrying out special research investigations for
master's theses. Staff members, in addition, teach at the
first three of these schools, and groups of students from

numerous other educational centers attend sessions at this center. Special service is given to the Newton public schools, and there is continual joint work on patients with the Children's Hospital, Massachusetts General Hospital, and Boston Dispensary. The senior director * of the center heads the board of trustees of the Boston Psychopathic Hospital. Among other things, he has collaborated with the American Law Institute in the planning of new legal processes for delinquent youth.

The researches of the Judge Baker Guidance Center are primarily dependent upon clinical service. Such laboratory work as is done is conducted by collaboration with other centers and is for clinical purposes. The center has its own library, with a half-time librarian, possesses most of the psychological and psychiatric periodical literature, and has, in addition, access to other library facilities of the city.

The studies now in progress at the center include standardization of norms of psychological tests and the development of improved apperception tests. Special attention is given to defects of visual perception. In another direction, case studies aim at a better understanding of the motivations of runaway boys, dynamic factors in general social antagonism in children, deficiencies in love experience and affectional capacity, and evaluation of citizenship training as part of a diagnostic and treatment service to juvenile delinquents. A special group of solitary delinquents is under special study, to elicit causative and contributing factors. Another study has to do with childhood "invention" tendencies and their connection with later paranoid tendencies, and still another is concerned with the pursuit of hobbies by young neurotics. One staff member is directing a continuous follow-up of a former Harvard Growth Study of a large number of children who are now in their twenties, to discover and study those who have become state wards. Workers from the National Youth

* Recently retired.

Administration have been assigned to assist in this rather extensive undertaking.

The co-directors of the center both divide their time equally between clinical work and research activity. Their studies, for which they have special staff aids, include, at the present time, an evaluation of the results of work done on past cases in order to determine the efficacy of treatment and the types of individual, treatment and therapist that have been effective or otherwise. Recently published is a study made, through visits to England, of the "Borstal System" of dealing with youthful offenders. A long-time research is also under way in the attempt further to clarify the issues presented by abnormal personalities, particularly the so-called psychopathic personalities.

The regular budget of the center provides for a certain amount of research time and assistance for the clinical staff. Funds for half-time research on the part of the directors have for several years been given equally by two donors.

CHICAGO, ILL.

University of Chicago

> *Division of Biological Sciences*
> *Otho S. A. Sprague Memorial Institute*
> *Orthogenic School*

Northwestern University
Michael Reese Hospital
Loyola University
Cook County Psychopathic Hospital
Institute for Psychoanalysis

Psychiatric research in the *University of Chicago* involves several departments within the *Division of Biological Sciences,* which includes the medical school and some independent agencies. "The *Otho S. A. Sprague Memorial Institute* supports research in psychiatry conducted on a coöperative basis in several departments of the University in association with the Division of Psychiatry of the Department of Medicine. The close geographic and working association of medical and fundamental sciences gives exceptional advantages for the study of psychiatric problems, which ramify so widely into many special fields.'' *

The funds (approximately $60,000 per annum) received by the University from the Institute are administered by a committee consisting of the dean of the division of biological sciences, the director of the university clinics, the director of the Otho S. A. Sprague Institute and the head of the division of psychiatry.

The research activities of the division of psychiatry fall into three classes. These include (1) clinical studies conducted with patients available in the clinics for both adults and children; (2) laboratory studies under the various departments; (3) collaborative research between staffs of the different departments. Some 40 to 50 projects are continuously in progress. While these cover a wide range of interests, there are special emphases, as in studies devoted to migraine, anxiety states, pre-psychotic symptoms and gastro-intestinal reactions; endocrine studies directed particularly toward gonadal and related functions; the action of ergotamine; experimental studies of emotions, through neurological, pharmacological and psychological approaches; behavior studies in cases of brain lesion, psychological studies of fantasy, applications of the meaning of the Rorschach and other mental tests under various clinical conditions; and studies of cerebral-electrical phenomena.

Coöperation is anticipated with sociology, education and law in regard to research problems of mutual interest to these fields and to psychiatry. The division of psychiatry already has teaching and coöperative relationships with the department of sociology and with the schools of social service administration, nursing and law, and it has a close informal relationship with the Chicago Institute for Psychoanalysis. A member of the psychiatric staff is assigned

---

* Quoted from an Announcement of the University of Chicago.

to pediatrics, and two members of the staff hold appointments to the Cook County Psychopathic Hospital.

There is interest in securing funds to extend the investigations into the sociological aspects of psychiatry and the community aspects of mental hygiene.

Unusual laboratory facilities are available at this center, as are also the rich library resources of the whole university. The in-patient psychiatric service admits about 160 cases yearly and consists of 11 beds for private patients. This clinical facility is exceptionally well staffed. All members of the staff are engaged in research, which is the primary objective, and they are selected with that function in view. About half their time is available for research, most of which is carried out under the Sprague Institute. They have contributed extensively to the scientific literature of psychiatry.

The *Orthogenic School* is a department of the University of Chicago responsible directly to the central administration. Its function is to provide for the study and treatment of children who have serious problems of behavior. It serves as one of the teaching resources for students of psychology and education, it conducts a course in child development, and it has responsibility for the field work of students from the School of Social Service Administration. The children are studied in part through the medical school and they may attend the university schools. They are referred by physicians, social agencies, schools and parents in the community. They are in general under 14 years of age.

The institution has a capacity of 34 in-patients, and a few patients (less than a dozen) are in transition, either in anticipation of admission or in process of being discharged. Quite a few of the children are schizophrenic cases and practically all are psychiatric cases. The activities include educational, social and therapeutic work. The staff consists of a director trained in education, psychology and psychiatry, a psycho-physiologist, a psychologist, two nurses, four teachers and three social supervisors. There is also an attending pediatrician.

The library facilities of the Orthogenic School are centralized with those of the University. The laboratories within the school are for physiologists and psychologists. They are equipped with electroencephalographic and polygraphic apparatus and will shortly have apparatus for electric shock treatment. Until now metrazol has been used.

The research interests of the school center on frustration and its physiological and psychological effects, and their relations to developed conditions of neuroses and psychoses. The research is both the result of individual interest and of staff projects and includes also the thesis problems of graduate students.

Northwestern University's department of neurology and psychiatry, operating under a common chairman, is a part of the division of medicine. It is closely affiliated with the Institute of Neurology, established in 1928 and widely recognized for its researches. With the department of physiology and other departments, the department of neurology and psychiatry contributes to the publications of the Institute and to its seminars and shares in its researches. It is closely related to the department of neuro-surgery. The plans of the medical school call for a special neuropsychiatric hospital to house neurology, neurosurgery and psychiatry.

By interlocking appointments from the faculties of pediatrics, clinical child guidance, otology and ophthalmology, these departments are more intimately bound into the work in neurology and psychiatry. Representatives from other departments act as liaison officers between members of the department of neurology and psychiatry in the out-patient clinic. Coöperative agreements exist also with the departments of anatomy, physiology, pathology, experimental medicine and surgery, all leading to reciprocal teaching and investigation.

Certain other schools and departments of the university are likewise in touch with the department of neurology and psychiatry, at times in an advisory capacity, at times for mutual teaching, and at times in carrying out treatment and research. Among these may be mentioned the School of Liberal Arts, the School of Law, the School of Dentistry, and the departments of psychology, sociology and speech.

The clinical material for teaching and research is obtained from the out-patient department, 75 per cent of whose patients are referred by social agencies, courts and other hospitals; from the Cook County, Wesley Memorial, Evanston, and Passavant Memorial Hospitals, all of which are part of the university hospitals; and from St. Luke's, Children's Memorial, and Michael Reese Hospitals which, in one way or another, are affiliated with the university.

The Cook County Psychopathic Hospital affords the most extensive material for teaching and research. Members of the faculty are employed in the psychopathic laboratory of the Cook County Criminal Court, the Municipal Court, and the Institute for Juvenile Research, and there they conduct research in collaboration with the department of neurology and psychiatry.

A number of the members of the faculty, some of whom are enrolled in the Graduate School, are employed by the Elgin State Hospital, Kankakee State Hospital, and at times other state hospitals, and research is conducted jointly by such state hospitals and the department. A similar relationship exists with the laboratory for neuropathology of the Cook County Hospital.

There is available to the department of neurology and psychiatry a suite of rooms arranged for research. These are fully equipped for study and research in neuropathology and neurophysiology, and partly for chemistry, and further equipment is available through the departments of physiology, chemistry, experimental medicine, the laboratory for surgical research, especially for animal experimentation, and other departments. Although adequately equipped for the present, the small research unit now at the department's disposal can and will be enlarged as appropriations and, particularly, the availability of good research workers warrant.

As stated above, the department of nervous and mental diseases of Northwestern University Medical School operates under the direction of a common chairman for both divisions. As a result, there is no differentiation between diseases of the nervous system that produce psychic disturbances and those that produce disturbances of the reflexes, sensation, motion, etc. Research is directed toward elucidation of functions and dysfunctions of the nervous system, and certain members of the faculty who are more interested in psychiatry are doing investigative work in pure physiology, while those with greater preoccupation in neurology are engaged in work on psychology. Consequently, no attempt is made to separate forms of research directed primarily toward psychiatry from those dealing exclusively with organic neurology.

An indication of the diversity of research interests may be seen from the titles of papers with psychiatric implications published during the last few years. Physiological investigations, for example, have considered effects of laughter on muscle tone, comparison of viscosity of muscles in catatonic and Parkinsonian rigidity, physiology of hyperpyrexia, heat regulation in chronic encephalitis, galvanic skin reflex and blood pressure reactions in the psychoneuroses.

Chemical studies have dealt with sodium amytal, effects of oxygen consumption rôle in the psychoses, hydrogen ion concentration, potassium and calcium during metrazol-induced convulsions in man, metabolic and chemical studies in Huntington's Chorea, and insulin tolerance in dementia praecox. Structural pathology has received attention in such studies as pathology of Huntington's Chorea, Pick's Disease, and tuberous sclerosis. Experimental pathology has been followed in studies of histopathologic changes in the brain in experimental hyperinsulinism, and the effect of insulin and metrazol on the central nervous system of animals.

Psychological and psychobiological studies include strephosymbolia, a study of scatter in the Stanford Binet test, suicide, psychoanalysis of manic depressive psychosis, psychopathology of tuberculosis, studies in affective psychology, trauma and invalid reactions, and psychoanalytic interpretation of a schizophrenic psychosis.

Clinical psychiatric investigations have dealt with neuropsychiatry in obstetrics and gynecology, a study of phobias, the relation of hereditary factors to prognosis in dementia praecox, psychiatric features of convalescence, and mental disturbance of chronic epidemic encephalitis.

Treatment has been a major concern in studies involving treatment of neurosyphilis, endocrine therapy in the psychoses, fever treatment in paresis, prolonged sleep therapy in psychoses, treatment of symptomatic psychoses occurring during pregnancy, studies in insulin treatment, and metrazol therapy in functional psychoses.

In 1935 a grant of $8,333.31 was made available to the department for epilepsy. A report of the work done under this project has been published in book form. Work in this field has continued since then with the same productiveness, although only a small portion of this fund has been allocated to Northwestern University Medical School.

With the exception of the intensive study of epilepsy, research and study has not been directed into special channels. It has been considered preferable to allow each man to attack a problem in which he develops a special interest. The research, therefore, is diversified. The reason for this is obvious. Until the university possesses a psychiatric hospital directly under its control, long-term, well-planned fundamental research is difficult.

Michael Reese Hospital is a voluntary general hospital, with an in-patient and out-patient psychiatric service that has for years served as a research and professional training center. Its research is supported by the Jewish Charities, by community funds and by private subscription. Many scientific contributions from this center have been reported in the psychiatric literature. The in-patient service has a capacity of 18 psychiatric beds and there is a well organized out-patient department. The staff consists of à chairman, who spends half-time at the hospital; four full-time psychiatrists, including a director of psychiatric services and two residents; five attending physicians; one intern; two psychologists; three psychiatric social workers; and seven clinic physicians. Some ten psychiatric social workers from the University of Chicago receive field training here. There are also two speech correction teachers.

Through inter-staff appointments there are connections with many other hospitals and with the medical schools of Chicago, in two of which teaching is carried on by psychiatrists from Michael Reese Hospital. It works closely also with the Chicago Institute for Psychoanalysis on psychosomatic problems. The hospital has an exceptional library, and two laboratories which are devoted to research, one neuropsychiatric and the other psychological.

The researches of this center include studies of electrical potential in the hypothalamus during emotional change, in schizophrenia, in epilepsy (in conjunction with Rorschach reactions) and in depressions, (in conjunction with shock treatments). Studies in the psychotherapy of behavior problems in childhood and adolescence follow psychoanalytic lines and include direct psychotherapy. School phobias in children are a subject of special interest. Psychological studies are concerned with variations in gastric secretion, correlated with personality types, psychological aspects of hyperventilation in childhood, and general studies of Rorschach techniques. Neurological studies are directed toward studies of emotion in chronic encephalitis and the effects of cerebral anoxia experimentally induced in dogs.

Psychiatric research at the *Loyola University* Medical School is dependent in part upon the biochemical laboratory facilities of the medical school, and in part upon the proximity of *Cook County Psychopathic Hospital*. This hospital also accommodates students of Northwestern and Rush Medical Colleges. It has an admission service for 170 patients, with a medical staff of nine psychiatrists, including six residents, two interns and a neuropathologist. There are also eight attending and associate psychiatrists, representing the various schools of psychiatry, and tying the hospital informally to most of the other institutions in the city. There is also a social service staff. Extensive consultation service is provided to the other departments of Cook County Hospital, and the psychiatric service receives, for neuropathological study, nervous tissue from autopsies of the hospital as a whole. It depends upon the clinical laboratories of the hospital for most of its clinical adjunct work.

Researches at Cook County Hospital largely follow individual interest and initiative. Attention has been particularly directed toward the use of guanadin and other substances in the treatment of schizophrenic patients and in producing remissions in other types of mental disorder.

Researches at Loyola Medical School are under the direction of a widely known contributor to the treatment of dementia praecox and look toward the isolation and application of anti-insulin hormones that seem to prevail in dementia praecox. All forms of biochemical and animal experimentation can, however, be carried on. Clinical material for such studies is available at the Cook County Hospital, and the director of research holds a research appointment at that hospital. The same is true of St. Luke's Hospital, which has a capacity of 22 psychiatric beds and in which the professor of psychiatry also holds an appointment.

Teaching connections include Loyola's own Mercy Hospital, with its nursing school, Holy Cross Hospital, and St. Francis Hospital, in Evanston. The director also teaches at the School of Nursing of the University of Chicago. Students from the School of Social Work of Loyola University receive both formal lectures and field training through the department of psychiatry and its affiliated services.

Loyola conducts a regular out-patient department in which social service facilities are available. The psychiatric department has some library facilities in the medical school, but depends chiefly upon the Crear Library, in which there is a file of all the medical libraries in the city and which has arrangements for the exchange of books.

The Institute of Psychonanalysis is a voluntary corporation that provides clinical service to patients; training in psychoanalysis to psychiatrists interested in acquiring proficiency in this field; and educational service to physicians, social workers, educators, social scientists, and others seeking to enlarge their professional foundations. The Institute has maintained a leading position in these respects, as is evident from its continuous contributions to scientific literature. Research in its field is usually difficult because of the small number of cases that can be handled by one person. This limitation has been offset to a considerable extent, however, through coöperative investigation by the dozen or so staff members of the Institute, and the effectiveness of the organization has been similarly enhanced by centering attention on a limited range of problems.

Contributing to its effectiveness is the extensive coöperation of the Institute with research and training centers in other fields. Psychiatrists trained at the Institute hold posts in general and mental hospitals, sanitaria, out-patient and clinic departments, state and county institutions, medical schools, and universities throughout the country. For purposes of clinical service, teaching, and further research, staff members of the Institute hold posts as clinical associates in hospitals, social agencies, and medical schools. Through this training and through participation of the

staff in the service of other agencies, the Institute enlarges
the scope of its work in the fields of psychiatry, medicine,
education, social service, and the social sciences. The institute has its own adjunct laboratory and a well equipped
psychoanalytic library.

The research activities of the Institute center primarily
around the interrelationships between emotional tensions
and resulting physiological changes which appear as
organic symptoms (psychosomatic research or vegetative
neuroses). It is widely recognized that the stresses and
strains of life frequently result in emotional tensions that
disturb the body system sufficiently to produce organic
symptoms. Efforts are made to reveal the specific connections, to determine exactly what emotional tensions
are involved and why they eventuate in the particular
physiological disturbance.

The first major group project consisted of an investigation of the specific emotions related to functional symptoms
of the gastrointestinal tract, particularly nervous colitis,
constipation, and disturbances resulting in peptic ulcers. A
similar group study was recently made of asthma, and there
are continuing studies of functional cardiac disorders,
particularly essential hypertension. Also in progress is a
study of the interrelationships between psychological and
hormonal changes in women during the menstrual cycle,
as well as investigations of psychological factors in other
endocrine and metabolic disturbances and in skin disease.
In addition, investigations are under way on relationships
between spirograms and emotional trends in the personality, and also psychological correlations with electroencephalograms, which have been taken annually for the
last five years. A grant from the Mary W. Harriman
Trust Fund has recently made possible a study of the
psychological factors in glaucoma.

For several years, the Institute has been experimenting
with the application of psychoanalytic principles to brief
forms of psychotherapy. Special funds made available
for this study in 1941 have made possible concentrated

and systematic investigation in this field which is expected to increase the direct clinical service of the Institute as well as to put psychoanalytic knowledge to work in the service of general psychiatric practice.

The research of the Institute is supported by a grant from the Rockefeller Foundation, by contributions from individuals, and by income from tuition and patients' fees. A five-year fellowship grant from the Rockefeller Foundation is devoted to the training of psychiatrists who hold teaching or research posts and who plan to continue in institutional work.

CINCINNATI, O.

University of Cincinnati
Cincinnati General Hospital
Jewish Hospital

> *Child Guidance Home*
> *May Institute for Research*

Children's Hospital
Longview State Hospital

Psychiatric research has received only scant attention in Cincinnati in the past. Recently, however, there has been a surge of interest arising from several sources.

The community facilities for psychiatric research are many and varied and there is an excellent spirit of coöperation. In the College of Medicine of the University of Cincinnati, the departments of biochemistry, anatomy, pharmacology, physiology and several others have laboratories that are well equipped for research work. These are intimately connected with the Cincinnati General Hospital, which also includes clinical laboratories in its medical, psychiatric and surgical departments. The Jewish Hospital, which is adjacent to Cincinnati General Hospital and the medical school, includes, in addition to its Child Guidance Home and the May Institute for Research, many opportunities and extensive equipment for research. The Children's Hospital, in the same vicinity, has research facilities well equipped for special approaches to psychiatric problems. The University of Cincinnati, through its psychology department and through the graduate school, also offers much equipment for research. Longview State Hospital, with a population of 2,800 psychiatric patients, has close ties with the medical school and offers not only a vast number of patients, but good facilities for chemical, electroencephalographic and clinical therapeutic research. Each of these centers has library facilities, the central library being in the Cincinnati General Hospital.

All these various means are used by interested individuals in an ever-changing relationship. The selection of loci of work depends sometimes on a desire to make use of available equipment and sometimes on the availability of patients. The coöperation is increasingly better and, although the research is planned, financed and carried out individually, there is much well-coördinated effort. A brief review of the approaches of the various groups will show this and will probably give the best indication of the direction of effort and the type of work in progress in Cincinnati.

At the College of Medicine of the *University of Cincinnati,* in the department of anatomy, neuropathologic examinations are made on some 600 to 700 brain specimens a year from the Cincinnati General Hospital, Hamilton County Hospital for Chronic Diseases, Cincinnati Tuberculosis Hospital, and Longview Hospital. Routine clinical and pathological correlations are made in these cases and certain of them are selected for further and more detailed anatomical and clinical correlations. This department has been especially interested in the last few years in the representation in the central nervous system of visceral, metabolic and emotional functions. Its studies of sugar metabolism and of the hypothalamic region of the brain are onstanding. The biochemical department has given particular attention to tissue changes correlated with psychoses. The department of physiology has worked closely with Longview Hospital on human behavior in relation to infections and endocrinological factors. The pharmacology department is likewise collaborating with Longview Hospital in investigating the pharmaco-dynamics of drugs used therapeutically in psychiatry. The department of psychology of the university, also in collaboration with Longview, is carrying on personality studies of both normal and psychotic persons. Here there is a definite concentration of interest on studies of mental fatigue.

The *Cincinnati General Hospital,* which is the chief clinical resource of the medical school and which has an extensive interchange of staff appointments with the latter, has a number of projects on the relationship of Vitamin B deficiency to mental disorders. In the laboratory of neuropathology, experimental studies on cerebral circulation are in progress. A plan is under way to collaborate with Longview Hospital in the determination of blood flow differences in various psychiatric patients. This includes a study of the substances that alter cerebral blood flow. The department of neurology is studying the treatment of postencephalitic Parkinsonism. It is also studying the mode of action of metrazol, in collaboration with the department of physiology of the medical school.

The psychiatric service of this hospital, which has an admission rate of over 1,000 patients, coöperates with various laboratories. The head of this department is professor of psychiatry in the medical school. The work on the cerebral circulation has already been mentioned. In addition, studies on certain clinical and laboratory aspects of alcoholism are made in collaboration with the *May Institute,* and Longview State Hospital has assisted with the electroencephalographic aspects of this work. This department is assisting on studies of psychiatric states occurring in the nutritional disorders, particularly pellagra, and looking especially toward treatment. This work is in progress in the Hillman Hospital in Birmingham, Alabama. The Central Clinic, which is operated under the direction of the professor of psychiatry by the Community Chest at the Cincinnati General Hospital, provides diagnostic and therapeutic service and offers an important clinical resource.

The *Jewish Hospital* has a very active research organization, which is engaged in studies of the pituitary gland and of sleep, convulsions, cerebral and peripheral blood flow, avitaminosis, and alcohol in the blood stream.

The *Child Guidance Home,* located on the grounds of the Jewish Hospital, has long exhibited research interest and productivity. Its interests include studies of behavior disorders in children, their measurement in terms of intellectual and social deviations, and the rôle of endocrine factors.

The *Children's Hospital,* adjacent to the City Hospital, is developing a psychiatric department. Its research activities include studies of encephalitis and poliomyelitis, particularly as to etiology and the properties of viruses.

Longview State Hospital has been striving, in spite of its limited staff, to carry out research projects on such time as its staff can spare from routine work. In addition to making clinical material available to other nearby research centers, the research carried on at this hospital is directed into three main channels—biochemical, physiological and therapeutic. It has made studies of the action of dilantin, especially in psychomotor epilepsy; of nicotinic acid and thiamin, wine of belladonna and allied preparations in the post-encephalitic states; of oestrin, stilboestrol and various autonomic preparations. Electroencephalographic studies of various disorders, blood flow studies of peripheral and cerebral circulation, and bacteriological blood studies have been undertaken. Some psychological studies of fatigue and of the effects of insulin therapy have been reported. The action of several oxidative stimulants has also been studied, particularly methylene blue and pyocyanine. In the biochemical field, the most important studies deal with changes of blood adrenalin in the new shock therapies and in various mental states.

In addition to these outstanding medical organizations a number of social service groups and other agencies have much to offer in the way of facilities for psychiatric studies, and these are available as needed. A large psychological laboratory operates in the school system. The employment center makes careful personality studies of all applicants for work. A family consultation service with trained workers operates with the advice of psychiatrists, who function in close coöperation with the above and other local agencies. The Board of Education operates a home for maladjusted boys and girls under the advice of the Central Clinic.

CLEVELAND, O.

Western Reserve University
City Hospital
Cleveland Guidance Center

In one way or another psychiatric research in Cleveland involves a linkage with *Western Reserve University* School of Medicine. The main psychiatric resource of the city is at the City Hospital which serves both city and county as a psychiatric observation center, admissions usually being limited to ninety days. All members of the resident staff and those in higher positions have teaching appointments at the medical school. The psychiatric department of the medical school is practically centered at the *City Hospital*, where most of the teaching under this department is done. This hospital accommodates some 300 patients of all types, has four residents, one psychologist and one psychiatric social worker. It has a large out-patient department attended by many visiting neuropsychiatrists. There is also a tie with Lakeside Hospital, where a course in psychobiology is offered and the principles of psychological medicine or "liaison psychiatry" are applied.

The psychiatric department has laboratory facilities

sufficiently equipped to meet the clinical needs of patients and, in addition, engages in biochemical studies, particularly along serological lines. It employes a full-time technician. There is provision for electroencephalographic studies, and there is an inactive neuropathological laboratory for which necessary equipment has only recently been provided. The library facilities are concentrated in a large central library which serves the whole hospital, with a psychiatric section containing standard books and periodicals for students and staff.

In addition to its ties to Western Reserve University, this hospital provides affiliate psychiatric nursing training to 28 nursing schools. The psychiatric division is well integrated with the hospital, so as to facilitate collaborative studies between the various departments. It provides one month of psychiatric experience to interns rotating through the several departments of the hospital. There is provision also for the training of students from the school of social work.

Research studies are primarily clinical in nature. Special attention has been given to ways of "softening" the muscular violence of shock treatments. In this connection, the department works closely, though informally, with the University of Nebraska, in Omaha, where special facilities and techniques for shock therapies have been developed. The effects of erythroidin have been especially studied in this connection, as also the effects of pitressin as a producer of convulsions. A long-time study is under way to work out the genesis of cerebral changes in ageing, particularly through electroencephalographic recordings. Experimental use of metrazol in treatment, studies of affective elements in recurrent schizophrenic breakdowns, use of the brain block technique to test cerebral function before operations, and psychiatric follow-up of brain surgery cases represent continuing interests. Collateral studies grow out of special opportunities provided by chance cases. These studies are supported by special donations made to the hospital.

Occasionally the psychiatric department of the hospital offers clinical material for studies made by other departments of the university, such as those under the Brush Foundation, whose major concern is with the growth process generally, and which has also collaborated with the Institute for Psychoanalysis in Chicago.

The *Cleveland Guidance Center,* a Community Fund agency, has teaching connections with the departments of nursing, pediatrics and applied social sciences of Western Reserve University. It functions largely as an out-patient service though it performs an admitting function as well as being professionally responsible for the Children's Aid Society, a study and treatment center for maladjusted children. The Guidance Center provides the psychiatric and psychological service for this institution, and is staffed by two psychiatrists and one fellow, three psychologists and three social workers, in addition to students from Western Reserve School of Applied Social Science. It is a training center in child psychiatry for The National Committee for Mental Hygiene. It makes admission studies on every girl sent to the convent of the Good Shepherd by the court or on voluntary commitment. A Rorschach study of each of these provides special research material. The director is consultant to St. Anne's Maternity Home for unmarried mothers, where a psychologist from the clinic makes regular studies of the babies. While the facilities of this child guidance center are purely clinical, it has ready access to the Cleveland Medical Society and Western Reserve libraries, and has received technical assistance from the Cleveland Clinic, a private group medical service.

The research interests of the center are directed especially toward the physiological factors in behavior deviations, particularly those of a neurological, endocrine and autonomic nature, toward hereditary elements, and the experimental application of chemical balances to deficiencies in these fields. The center is engaged at the present time in a study of spastic children, jointly with the Association for the Crippled and Disabled.

LOUISVILLE, KY.

University of Louisville

Psychiatric researches in Louisville, Kentucky, are coordinated through the department of psychiatry of the University of Louisville School of Medicine. Besides teaching, consultation and research ties with all other departments in the medical school and other units of the University of Louisville, formal affiliations link the department closely with the City Hospital, Childrens Free Hospital, Louisville Mental Hygiene Clinic, and the observation center of the Louisville and Jefferson County Home (for children). All of these are practically adjacent to the university. Through inter-staff appointments and consultation services, working relationships have been established with numerous other state and local institutions and agencies.

The department of psychiatry is intimately linked with all other departments of the medical school through joint teaching, in which the patient as a whole is considered along with his organ pathology, and joint studies frequently grow out of this close association. Teaching of physical diagnosis, for example, is accompanied by study of the patient as a person. The City Hospital provides clinical opportunities, both in-patient and out-patient, for the medical school and is its chief clinical resource, affording some 45 beds for psychiatric cases of all types and a daily out-patient service. The hospital has a staff of three full-time psychiatrists, a full-time resident, one senior and two junior interns, and two psychiatric social workers. It has, in addition, several part-time workers and a visiting staff. The psychiatric in-patients studied by junior students are followed up in the senior year, wherever they may be. The screening service, both in- and out-patient, serves to bring psychiatric cases to attention very early and on positive indications.

The Mental Hygiene Clinic, which especially serves children, is under the same direction as are the psychiatric activities of the City Hospital and the psychiatric teaching at the medical school. It has also a fellow in child psychiatry from The National Committee for Mental Hygiene, a psychologist and three psychiatric social workers. It serves practically all of the community agencies—schools, courts, etc.—that are interested in the problems of children and offers opportunities for research. The library facilities of the whole complex of psychiatric services in Louisville are likewise interchangeable and cross-indexed. They include the small libraries of the psychiatric department of the Mental Hygiene Clinic and the general library of the City Hospital, which serve also the clinical classes of the medical school, and the large central library of the medical school, located two blocks from the hospital. These libraries include some 30 current neurological, psychiatric and mental hygiene periodicals, as well as back files of periodicals in these and related fields.

While practically all of the researches reported under way in this center are clinical in nature, they are occasionally supported by laboratory studies. Advantage is taken of chance opportunities in clinical cases to make special studies, albeit there is a continuous thread of enduring interests running through the investigative activities. Investigation of functions of the frontal lobe, through the psychiatric study of surgical cases, reflects a collaboration between the departments of psychiatry and surgery. Similarly, psychological studies in cardio-vascular cases, to determine psychosomatic elements in failure or non-failure, reflect a collaboration with internal medicine. Encephalographic studies of younger and older problem and delinquent children aim toward clarifying the genesis of correlated changes of electric potential.

On the preventive side, continuous experimentation is involved in efforts to educate foster mothers and nurses in the care of dependent and sick children. Sub-shock treatment of psychoneurotics is limited to insulin, while both insulin and metrazol treatment are the subject of a long-time follow-up study of patients. A continuing study, combining laboratory and clinical work, includes routine bromide serological determinations. An attempt to understand judgmental defects of general paretics is based upon experimental hypnosis. Experimental work in the psychiatric education of medical students is directed particularly toward treatment. A psychiatric fellow serves as consultant to the pediatric out-patient service of the medical school and City Hospital and aids in teaching.

The observation center of the Louisville and Jefferson County Home employs a full-time psychiatrist who has teaching and research connections with the medical school as well as close ties with the other county facilities for children.

Psychiatric connections with other departments of the university are effected chiefly through mental hygiene courses given in the departments of social service administration, dentistry and public health and nursing, while the student health service of the university receives clinical consultation service. Outside the university, lectures are given at the Southern Baptist and Presbyterian Seminaries. A routine psychiatric study was undertaken of all admissions to the House of the Good Shepherd following a survey by the clinical psychologist. Consultation is also given to the Kings Daughters Home for incurables (all ages), the Lakeland State Hospital, some of whose staff serve in the out-patient department, the United States Marine Hospital, and the Kosair Hospital for Crippled Children. A close relation with the U. S. Public Health Service Hospital for drug addicts (Lexington) brings the advice of their psychiatrists into the research program in a valuable way. Relations are also maintained with the practicing physicians of the community to whom consultation service is provided as a part of university policy.

While the laboratory facilities under psychiatric direction are limited to bromide determination and electroencephalography, the clinical adjunct and research facilities of the whole complex of institutions in this center are freely exchanged and extensively used, particularly in cardiological studies, in which personal evaluations are also made. There are, in other words, excellent psycho-somatic resources, both clinical and experimental.

NEW HAVEN, CONN.

Yale University

Medical School
Clinic of Child Development
Institute of Human Relations

New Haven Hospital

Psychiatric Service in the Community

Psychiatric research in New Haven is the expression of a complex of facilities, including those of *Yale University* and various New Haven agencies. Much of the work reported both from the department of psychiatry in the *Medical School,* whose primary function is teaching and clinical service, and from the Clinic of Child Development, which is concerned particularly with research, is the expression of an effort that extends outward into these community agencies or inward from them.

The *Clinic of Child Development* is so well known for its many scientific contributions that no evidence of this need be presented here. Its systematic researches are designed to chart the patterns and stages of normal behavior development in the first years of life. Clinical and experimental studies deal with deviations and special aspects of development, such as mental defects in infancy, cerebral palsies, endocrine disorders, pre-maturity, reading disabilities, laterality, resemblances in twins, etc. Service is rendered to a score of community agencies and also to university departments by the examination of children under consideration for adoption and those presenting developmental defects and deviations. A "guidance nursery" which provides for four different age groups is used for the study and treatment of personality problems.

The staff of the clinic includes psychological, neurophysiological, and pediatric personnel, a medical extern and a technician. It makes extensive use of the cinema as a recording device for preserving the evidences of human behavior and making detailed studies of it in terms of maturity and individuality. The clinic has its own library as well as ready access to the other libraries of Yale University. It has also a photographic research library with an extensive, well catalogued collection of films delineating normal and atypical development. The clinic offers instruction and opportunity for individual study with facilities for observation (by one-way vision) to pediatric students and students in the School of Nursing.

The researches within the department of psychiatry at Yale reflect a wide range of interest. There are basic scientific studies, including studies of chemical changes in the blood (urobilinogen, iodine, and serum lipoids); peculiarities and differences of physiological and psychological functions; and special attention is given the functions of respiration, sleep, metabolism, nutrition, motor activity, speed, perception, persistence of effort, and old age, middle age, and immaturity; to certain clinical types: organic disorders, speech and reading disabilities, and to various personality types. There are also various electroencephalographic studies.

On the clinical psychiatric side, research is directed toward the effects of sedatives, differentiations of headache, the handling of personal problems of prospective parents, post-partum personality disorders, and psychosomatic medicine. On the sociological side, plans are in process for a study of attitudes of families towards commitment to mental hospitals. In addition, there are a number of projects in experimental and clinical psychology. For many years special attention has been given also to psychiatric needs of college students. Methods of psychiatric teaching have likewise been given special consideration. There is clearly an unusual emphasis in this center on social psychiatry.

The department of psychiatry is well equipped with laboratory facilities and has recourse to such facilities in other departments. There is abundant evidence of research productivity both by individual workers and by the various administrative units referred to above. Some 10 or 11 persons are conducting researches directly related to the department of psychiatry. It also has its own library.

While administratively independent of Yale University, the *New Haven Hospital* is functionally inseparable from it and is the site of many activities closely identified with Yale Medical School. Integrated with it is an in-patient psychiatric service of 50 beds, which is functionally a part of the department of psychiatry of Yale. It is well staffed and slow enough in turnover to allow for careful recording, continued study and treatment, and complete service from pre-admission study to follow-up. It houses the psychiatric out-patient clinic which offers traditional psychiatric services to the community, and is also the headquarters of another clinic, namely, *Psychiatric Service in the Community,* which is supported by the Community Fund through the local mental hygiene society. This provides a consultation service to community agencies at their own respective headquarters. The staff of the former is largely assigned from the department of psychiatry and some of the staff of the latter have appointments in that department. It is making special prenatal studies in coöperation with the department of obstetrics and gynecology.

Elsewhere within the university there are other resources and interests that strengthen the two main foci of research in human behavior. Within the medical school the divisions of physiological chemistry, neurological surgery, medical neurology, internal medicine, pediatrics, obstetrics and gynecology at one time or another have collaborated on research. There is a neurological study unit that meets regularly and that coöperates with the department of psychiatry. This linkage is further strengthened by the consultation service given to these departments both by the department of psychiatry and by the Clinic of Child

Development. There is unusual interest within the department of public health on problems of human behavior, and the *Institute of Human Relations* has a staff especially qualified for this type of research.

Members of the special psychological staff of the department of psychiatry have appointments also in the department of psychology, and the department of psychiatry provides instruction to the Schools of Nursing, Law and Divinity.

Within the community are several other agencies that are doing a high grade of technical work, which benefits greatly from their proximity to Yale University, and that in turn contribute abundantly to the research potentialities of this center by virtue of their practical service. Here again in several instances there are overlapping appointments. Noteworthy among these are the Connecticut Society for Mental Hygiene and its New Haven branch, which have a close relationship to the department of psychiatry, and the Children's Community Center which provides unusual facilities for the individual study of children on a residential basis. The interlockings of all these various resources in New Haven are so intricate that any attempt to describe them here would be inadequate.

PHILADELPHIA, PA.

University of Pennsylvania

School of Medicine
Graduate School of Medicine

Pennsylvania Hospital

Institute of the Pennsylvania Hospital

Philadelphia General Hospital
Jefferson Medical College
Temple University School of Medicine
Gladwyne Colony
Elwyn Training School
Philadelphia Child Guidance Clinic

Philadelphia's long leadership in neurology and psychiatry has brought about an interlocking of its various centers to such a degree that they cannot be adequately interpreted separately. The complex of research and educational activities in this city involves the University of Pennsylvania School of Medicine and Graduate School of Medicine, Department for Mental and Nervous Diseases of the Pennsylvania Hospital, Philadelphia General Hospital, Jefferson Medical College, Temple University School of Medicine, Gladwyne Colony, Philadelphia Child Guidance Clinic, and others.

The *University of Pennsylvania* and the *Pennsylvania Hospital,* although separate corporate institutions, are especially close and are formally linked together through the graduate and undergraduate vice-deanship and professorship, respectively, of two members of the hospital staff. Many others of the staff have appointments at the university. At the same time, some members of this hospital's staff have appointments at the Jefferson and Woman's Medical Colleges. The Philadelphia General Hospital is an important teaching adjunct of the University of Pennsylvania School of Medicine, as well as other medical schools, and has on its visiting staff the director of the Gladwyne Colony, who also holds a University of Pennsylvania appointment. The director and other staff members of the Philadelphia Guild Guidance Clinic have appointments at the University of Pennsylvania, cither through the medical school or the Pennsylvania School of Social Work. A similar close relationship exists between the University of Pennsylvania and Friends Hospital and Elwyn Training School. The psychiatric faculties of Temple University School of Medicine and Jefferson Medical College have appointments also at the Philadelphia General Hospital.

Researches at the Pennsylvania Hospital, which has a long-standing reputation for scientific contributions in the psychiatric field, must be considered jointly with the University of Pennsylvania, because the intimate relationship between the two permits of mutual availability of most of the personnel and of library, laboratory and other resources of both. The professor of neurology of Jefferson Medical College and the professor of psychiatry at Woman's Medical College are staff members of the Pennsylvania Hospital. This hospital has patients in two departments. In one there is a psychotic population of 190, with 238 yearly admissions; in the other there is a neurotic population of 50. The *Institute of the Pennsylvania Hospital,* a special unit established for experimental study in mental hygiene, is an integral part of this center, in which much of the research is conceived and brought to fruition.

Recently, a member of the department of psychiatry of the University of Pennsylvania, who is also associated with the Institute of the Pennsylvania Hospital and the Philadelphia General Hospital, has been appointed professor of psychiatry at the Woman's Medical College. This completes a practical working organization of teaching and clinical facilities embracing four medical schools, an acute and chronic public psychiatric hospital, a leading private mental hospital, an institute for psychoneurotic patients, out-patient clinics, general and special laboratories, and many other resources.

The Pennsylvania Hospital conducts special laboratories in biochemistry and electro-physics, in addition to those needed for clinical service. It has a well equipped library of books and periodicals, which is maintained by sizeable appropriations. It has received frequent grants from various foundations for the support of its researches. It has published some 150 articles in the past three years.

Some of the studies and experiments conducted at the Pennsylvania Hospital and the University of Pennsylvania are undertaken at intervals as timely opportunities present themselves, some follow the current interests of individual staff members, while others represent a continuing orientation. Clinical studies include critical evaluations of shock therapies and psychotherapeutic procedures, follow-up evaluations of longitudinal studies, and studies of psychosomatic problems. Clinical, psychological, neurological and pharmacological studies, involving laboratory determinations, represent a rather continuous trend and include blood chemistry and intra-cranial pressure studies, animal experiments, electrocardiographic studies, and studies of the action of dilantin, carbon disulphide and delvinol. A closely controlled study of a promising remedy for migraine is in progress. Provision has also been made for researches into tissue metabolism. Worthy of note is the work done in the facilities available for the study of brain and nerve potentials. Psychological studies deal with vocational selection and guidance, changes accompanying treatment, and educational capacities. Language and speech difficulties in children are the subject of special attention. There are also researches in social psychiatry, particularly in relation to mass reactions.

The *Philadelphia Child Guidance Clinic* has a similar close connection with the University of Pennsylvania. It has contributed continuously to the field of child psychiatry, through its clinical studies, through the elucidation of psychological growth, and the dynamics of therapeutic work with children.

The *Philadelphia General Hospital,* with a bed capacity for approximately 300 patients and with 4,500 admissions yearly, is essentially a municipal receiving hospital which provides some continued treatment service. It has a large intake of acute and chronic psychiatric cases. Also available to it for study is the large amount of clinical material represented by the approximately 5,000 patients at the Philadelphia State Hospital. In addition, it conducts an out-patient neuropsychiatric clinic, to which over 1,000 patients were admitted during 1941. On its visiting staff are appointees of every medical school in the city. Its close contacts with leaders who have other connections in the city expose it constantly to varied influences and renders its rich clinical material available to research centers. Unfortunately, its budget allows of no formal research program of its own, in spite of the unparalleled combination of scientists on its visiting staff, but it is a meeting ground for those interested in research and is used extensively as a teaching resource by the University of Pennsylvania, which is adjacent to it, and by other schools of medicine. It has an enviable autopsy record, but its laboratories are at present limited to clinical service. Its senior attending psychiatrist is director of the Gladwyne Colony, which depends, in part, upon the clinical material of the Philadelphia General Hospital for its researches.

Gladwyne Colony is a proprietary institution of 80 beds, with a long-standing interest in research. It has centered its attention for years upon biochemical changes, particularly those of the blood. The determinations of globulin and albumin are routine practice with all patients, so that a large body of data has been built up. Continuous attention is also given to studies of capillary habitude of various types of psychiatric patients.

Elwyn Training School is a voluntary institution for mental defectives, with a capacity of some 1,090 patients. It also receives many state patients. Its research activities fluctuate and are carried out from time to time in relation to other centers, such as the University of Pennsylvania or the Philadelphia General Hospital. The research is under the general direction of the superintendent and is carried on largely by one staff member whose current investigation has to do with the metabolism of patients with mongolism, and with immunology. Studies of the therapeutic and educational value of music and its influence on mental and social development receive special attention.

The *Jefferson Medical College* Hospital, through its psychiatric department, conducts psychiatric out-patient services for children and for adults, and also provides an active in-patient consultation service to the general wards of the hospital. The child psychiatric clinic functions in close affiliation with the pediatric department. Through a fellowship in psychiatry, active clinical research is conducted in psychosomatic medicine.

For teaching purposes, use is made of the facilities of the psychiatric department of the Philadelphia General Hospital, where the professor of psychiatry of Jefferson Medical College and several members of the Jefferson psychiatric staff hold major psychiatric appointments.

A close coöperative relationship exists between the Institute of the Pennsylvania Hospital and Jefferson Medical College through the sharing of a psychiatric fellow. The professor of psychiatry at Jefferson is an honorary consultant of the Institute, and other members of his staff also hold positions there.

Jefferson Medical College has an unusually active neurological department which draws on the Philadelphia General Hospital and other local sources for its material. The researches of this center deal with problems of out-patient hypothalamic functions and emotions, anxiety neuroses, impotence and convulsions, and also with biochemical and physical studies of nervous function.

Psychiatric research at *Temple University School of Medicine* is limited by the lack of a psychiatric in-patient facility. However, a close relationship between the department of psychiatry and the psychiatric wards of the Philadelphia General Hospital affords potentialities far exceeding the present limited research activity. There is a psychiatric out-patient department.

The department of psychiatry is chiefly a teaching unit, but it also engages in research. The major research related to this field is conducted by the McCarthy Foundation, under which studies in experimental neurology and physicochemical studies are pursued. The laboratories are well equipped for the specific studies undertaken and have special resources for electroencephalographic, photographic, spectrographic and, by collaboration with the pathological laboratory, neuropathological work. There is an unusually well equipped shop where almost any type of apparatus may be made. The library facilities are fair but are richly supplemented by the library of the College of Physicians and Surgeons.

In the department of psychiatry electrocardiographic characteristics of acutely psychotic patients are under investigation. This department is also attempting to define the personality characteristics of failing students through the Rorschach test.

The work in experimental neurology includes animal studies in otoneurology, especially on the relation of labyrinth and cortex. Special attention is also given to studies in neurophthalmology similarly conceived.

The physicochemical studies consider especially the spinal fluid in convulsive states. Electrical conductivity and interferometric methods are used in these studies. Physicochemical studies of the spinal fluid are also made with reference to tabes and in insulin and metrazol treatment for psychoses. There is occasional interchange of scientific activity with the department of chemistry at Yale University, and with the Phipps Institute (for tuberculosis) in Philadelphia. Current studies include also measurements of the permeability of brain cells in convulsive disorders and under convulsants, anesthetics and hypnotics. Animal experimentation is employed in these studies. Studies of brain potentials are directed toward the discovery of the source and nature of these potentials. Studies of psychosomatic relations include experiments with picrotoxin-barbituate and bulbocapinine-benzedrine antagonisms, subthalamic lesions and their effect on sleep, and the cortical relations of the rage reaction.

The directors both of the experimental neurological and of the biochemical and physical studies have a long and respected record of research contributions before and during the ten years of their activity under the McCarthy Foundation.

ST. LOUIS, MO.

Washington University

Psychiatric research at Washington University centers in the department of neuropsychiatry, and involves not only other departments of the medical school and university, but various community institutions and agencies, such as Barnes Hospital, which is the general hospital associated with the medical school; the Washington University Clinics, which provide the out-patient service; the City Hospital and Bliss Psychopathic Hospital, whose services are shared with St. Louis University; the City Sanitarium for Chronic Mental Diseases; the Homer G. Phillips Hospital for Negroes; and the family and children's agencies of the city.

The department of neuropsychiatry has been recently organized independently of the department of medicine, which earlier carried this function. Even before the organization of the new department, research was carried on as far as limited financing and a part-time staff permitted, and worthy contributions were made to the scientific literature. The present administration is definitely research-minded. It includes professors or assistant professors of neurology, psychiatry and medical psychology on a full-time basis, a professor of clinical neurology and assistant professors and instructors on half-time, as well as appointees in other departments, such as pediatrics and sociology.

The department of pediatrics was one of the first in the country to assume psychiatric functions and it collaborates closely with the department of neuropsychiatry in the field of child psychiatry. It conducts a child guidance clinic whose scientific studies have been preoccupied with endocrinological and metabolic abnormalities in relation to mental states. It also works closely with the Children's Hospital.

The department of social work has a professor of psychiatry who also holds an appointment in the medical school and in the principal family and children's social agencies of the city. This department's investigative interests are directed particularly toward the analysis of the psychological processes involved in the common routine procedures of social agency function, such as the intake of cases. These studies are psychoanalytically oriented.

The psychiatric studies of the faculty of the department of neuropsychiatry have in the past tended, in part, toward the psychological problems of patients with organic disease as well as personal and situational elements in medical practice. Additions to the staff and equipment recently made with the aid of outside Foundations permit more detailed psychosomatic studies, particularly in relation to colitis and the allergies and the effects of modified interpersonal relations on neurotic and psychotic states. Previous studies have otherwise been largely neurological in nature and this interest persists in the present set-up.

Current clinical research interests are pointed toward psychosomatic studies and toward studies of interpersonal relations as they underlie psychoses and neuroses. The former studies involve combined physiological and interview techniques for the study of asthma and hypertension. The latter are directed toward therapy of the neuroses and psychoses and toward the available persons actively involved in the life problems of the patient.

Neuropsychological researches are directed toward the nervous system, with special reference to the processes of learning, memory and more complex adaptations. The rôle of the frontal lobes in affect and "experimental neuroses" in animals is studied through experiments on monkeys. An attempt is being made to adapt experimental psychological methods to neuropsychiatric problems, especially disorders associated with cerebral damage.

Barnes Hospital, located at the medical school, has beds for neurological cases available for psychosomatic studies. The Washington University Clinics provide the out-patient facility for the hospitals associated with the medical school.

Neurological and psychoneurotic cases are serviced here and provide case material for teaching and research. The City Hospital has a neurological ward of 60 beds, 30 of which are under the clinical direction of Washington University Medical School and 30 under St. Louis University Medical School. It has all the facilities for research except special research equipment.

The Bliss Psychopathic Hospital is the receiving hospital for the city's mental patients. It provides for adults and children, both colored and white. It has excellent research laboratories, and special observation facilities. Its 300 beds are divided as to teaching and research use between the two medical schools. The City Sanitarium for chronic mental disease has a less formal connection with the medical schools, but is available for research.

Laboratory facilities at Washington University Medical School are well supplied and fully equipped, together with animal quarters. There are neurophysiological laboratories and an equipment shop, electroencephalograph and full surgical equipment. The neuropathological laboratory is a joint facility of the departments of pathology, neurosurgery and neuropsychiatry.

SAN FRANCISCO, CAL.

Stanford University
University of California

> Medical School
> Institute of Child Welfare

California Department of Institutions

Stanford University Medical School conducts psychiatric research with respect both to children and to adults. The adult psychiatric work is performed in a separate department of psychiatry, which is engaged in numerous research projects, on its own and in collaboration with other departments of the university hospital, the medical school and other agencies. It has at its disposal an abundance of clinical material both in the psychiatric wards and in the out-patient services.

The hospital has 17 beds devoted to the study and treatment of patients who present mental disorders of one kind or another, and is staffed by two full-time psychiatrists in the adult division, and nine part-time or consultant staff members; one full-time psychiatrist and two part-time or consultant staff members in the child psychiatry division, with a complement of six graduate and seven student nurses, and four attendants. In the adult division there are one resident and two assistant residents in full-time service, and interns on the medical service of the hospital spend four months in the division, two interns being on service at a time. In addition to the 17 beds at Stanford Hospital, the division has charge of one-half the service at the San Francisco Hospital, where a 40 bed unit is functioning at the present time.

The division of child psychiatry is operated jointly by the pediatric and psychiatric departments. It is managed by a council represented by these two departments. It conducts a psychiatric clinic for children, both in-patient and out-patient, which is intimately connected with the university's department of psychology at Palo Alto and through which field work opportunities are afforded for the training of students in psychometrics, Rorschach testing, etc.

The laboratory facilities of the Stanford Medical School and hospitals are available to both divisions. These facilities permit the complete study of all patients as well as the pursuit of research projects from the standpoints of clinical pathology, biochemistry, bacteriology, pharmacology, physiology and electroencephalography. The personnel of these departments consists of the heads of those medical school divisions together with all necessary technical assistance. There is a growing library in the child psychiatry clinic, in addition to a fine collection of psychiatric books and periodicals at the Lane Library, which is part of the medical school.

The department of child psychiatry is of recent organization, but there are already evidences of active research interest and the beginnings of well formulated projects. Research work in progress reflects a special interest in the correlation of educational methods with the emotional problems of childhood. Recently published studies deal with reading disabilities, psychogenic factors in physical complaints, and children's reactions to crime and "horror" stories on the screen and the radio.

Researches in the division of adult psychiatry include studies of physiological changes associated with alcoholism, conducted in conjunction with the department of physiology and the State Department of Motor Vehicles; a study of psychoses associated with deafness, in collaboration with the department of otolaryngology; psychological studies of individuals with essential hypertension, undertaken in coöperation with the department of medicine and the student health service at Palo Alto; a similar study of ulcer patients, also with the aid of the department of medicine; a study of emotional influences in cases of atrophic dermatitis, in collaboration with the department of dermatology; studies of epilepsy, involving the experimental production of seizures in animals, and electroencephalographic studies on humans and animals; studies of anticonvulsants in association with the department of pharmacology; studies of the cause and treatment of pain in association with the departments of anatomy and neurosurgery; and an investigation of behavior syndromes and brain pathology produced in chicks with vitamin deficiencies.

Psychiatric research at the *University of California Medical School* is in the potential and formative rather than the actual stage and waits upon the completion of the Langley Porter Clinic, a state psychopathic hospital, now in the process of establishment on the medical school campus in San Francisco. With this new development there is anticipated a far-reaching program of psychiatric teaching and research which will greatly broaden and deepen the interests of the medical school in this field. This will involve a reorganization and expansion of the present activities in psychiatry, for which no separate department was previously provided in the medical school, the psychiatric staff being part of the department of medicine, so far as work with adults was concerned, with a separate staff of psychiatrists attached to the department of pediatrics for work with children. Both staffs have, nevertheless, been actively engaged in research work.

The Langley Porter Clinic is being built on land adjacent to the medical school and the University of California Hospital. It is expected that the building will be completed and ready for occupancy on July 1, 1942. There will be beds for 100 patients, including an 18-bed neurosurgical ward, and a 16-bed children's ward. There will be an out-patient department with 20 offices for psychiatrists, psychologists and psychiatric social workers. There will be a number of laboratory rooms with the usual equipment and a rather elaborate set-up for electroencephalography; also an operating room suite and an X-ray department. It is expected that neuropathology will be developed particularly in conjunction with the California state hospital system.

At this time the size and composition of the staff have not been completely determined. There will, however, be a close affiliation with the University of California Hospital in which interns, assistant residents and residents will spend a part of their time in psychiatry. There will also be an affiliation of the nursing students so that the student nurses will spend a period of two months in psychiatry. There will probably be 12 residencies in psychiatry open to graduates of Class "A" medical schools, who have had at least one year of general hospital training. Through affiliation with the University of California the services of a number of different departments will be utilized and courses of training given, including courses for psychiatric social workers and psychologists. Psychiatry will be taught to medical students during their second and fourth years at the Langley Porter Clinic and during the third year at the San Francisco Hospital.

The university library includes a large neuropsychiatric collection which will be housed in the new psychopathic hospital. The library, pronounced by the Council on Medical Education and Hospitals of the American Medical Association as one of the foremost collections possessed by a medical school, subscribes to several hundred current medical journals, including 32 psychiatric journals. In addition, there is a pathological museum containing much material on neuropathology.

Research interests at this center have been extensive and diverse, including, on the physiological side, studies in neurophysiology, biochemistry, biophysics, and psychophysiology, and on the pathological side, studies in neuroanatomy, bacteriology and immunology, pharmacology, neuropathology and psychopathology; and plans are being laid for a more concerted attack on problems in all these fields. There are currently in progress many special studies not characterized as formal research projects, but oriented toward such objectives as making psychiatric teaching more effective, acquainting students with the social and emotional components in all forms of illness, and arriving at more practical methods for the satisfactory examination of patients, recording of results, and shortening psychotherapeutic procedures applicable to a large psychiatric out-patient department. During the past year, special clinical demonstration studies in the administration of insulin and other shock therapies have been carried on in coöperation with the California Department of Institutions.

Recent research trends and interests are reflected in studies of such problems as: brain metabolism, with special reference to lipoids; blood brain permeability barriers, with special reference to convulsive phenomena; the phenomena of artificially induced increased cranial pressure in relation to refinements in clinical diagnostic procedure; alcoholism and the rôle of toxic agents versus psychological factors in the production of malignant psychic reactions; psychophysiological phenomena of anxiety with reference to hyperventilation and its associated altered metabolism; sodium chloride depletion in anxiety and allied states; and vitamin therapy in muscular dystrophy. A new research has just been organized for a study of the relationship of head injuries to personality disorders. This will be carried out in cooperation with the department of neurosurgery, the department of physiology, and the department of psychology at Berkeley. Both acute and chronic cases of head injuries will be studied from the neurological, psychiatric, psychological and neurophysiological approaches.

In child psychiatry, studies are in progress on such problems as alterations in personality and intellect in relation to a variety of physical diseases and disabilities; mental characteristics of deaf mutes; correlation between pneumoencephalographic findings and mental development; long-time investigations of children early described as psychopathic; and varieties of mental deviations found in juvenile delinquents.

Another focus of research activity at the University of California, but not connected with the medical school, is the *Institute of Child Welfare,* located at Berkeley. This is essentially a center for graduate study, with research interests involving various aspects of human growth and development. Staff members represent such specialized fields as psychology, physiology, anthropology, and statistics, and in several instances hold joint appointments in teaching departments in the university. The children selected for study attend the Institute nursery school and are included in various growth studies conducted in coöperation with local school systems; they are not clinic cases of the problem behavior variety, but represent, rather, the normal range of school children, dealt with from a broad psychobiological or biosocial point of view. The principal investigations include the following:

(1) The Berkeley Growth Study, begun in 1928, is con-

cerned with a series of problems involving mental, motor and physical development, in a group of children studied from birth to maturity. The program of psychological study is essentially descriptive, involving (a) the assessment, seriatim, of each individual's status in the group in a wide range of characteristics, (b) the study of trends and other variations in status, and (c) the analysis of certain correlated factors. While interest has not been directed primarily toward personality nor toward attempts at the detailed interpretation of growth dynamics, considerable use has been made of qualitative observations and of material from interviews, in addition to the more largely quantitative records.

(2) The Guidance Study, begun in 1930, has attempted (a) to trace the course of personality development and to investigate relationships between behavior patterns and such variables as physical growth, intellectual development and environmental influences; (b) to study specific behavior manifestations in normal children as compared with "problem" children; and (c) thus to determine why some individuals develop mature and sturdy personalities and others do not.

(3) The Growth Study of Adolescents, begun in 1932, has involved seriatim records, from the fifth through the twelfth grade, of (a) physical development, with special emphasis upon physiological changes during adolescence; and (b) psychological characteristics, as represented particularly in studies of social behavior and of interpersonal relationships in the adolescent "peer-culture."

The *California Department of Institutions,* at Sacramento, which has jurisdiction over the state institutions for the mentally ill and the mentally defective, is actively promoting psychiatric research in several directions. Coöperative relationships are maintained for this purpose with the University of California and the California Institute of Technology. The principal lines of investigation under way at the present time are in connection with the several shock therapies and in the field of psychiatric social service. Research in insulin coma and various convulsive types of therapy for schizophrenia and other psychoses is conducted under the direction of a member of the faculty of the University of California Medical School, with the collaboration of the medical staffs of the Camarillo, Stockton, and Patton State Hospitals. Studies of convulsive therapy, by means of electric shocks and of electronarcosis, are conducted mainly at the California Institute of Technology, upon experimental animals, and at Patton State Hospital in connection with clinical aspects. Studies in psychiatric social work are in progress in several state hospitals as part of the department's program for the extension of extramural care of mental patients. In addition, the director of the department has carried to completion a series of studies of mental disorders in twins, reports of which have been published.

For many years the Alhambra Sanatorium at Rosemead, California, has been the center of studies in heredity, carried on chiefly by its director. With his appointment to the directorship of the state department of institutions, this activity was transferred to the capital at Sacramento.

Case records secured from some 1,016 pairs of twins have been partially analyzed and classified according to indications of developing psychosis, epilepsy, mental deficiency and delinquency. Some studies of this material have already been published. In view of the developing department of psychiatry at the University of California, in close relationship with the central state psychopathic hospital, these studies may in the future also be a part of the research work of the University of California, as also will be the studies conducted by the various state hospitals. The extensive laboratory and other scientific resources of the University of California are being made available for collaboration. Already studies in insulin shock and other treatment procedures for schizophrenia are under way.

CHAPTER VII
Reports of Individual Centers

ALBANY, N. Y.

New York State Department of Mental Hygiene

THE conduct of psychiatric research has long been a major function of this department, which is responsible for the maintenance of the 26 institutions for the mentally ill, mental defectives and epileptics, that comprise the New York state hospital system. The clinical research and general scientific activities of the department are centralized in the New York State Psychiatric Institute and Hospital, Columbia Medical Center, New York City, which is charged under the state's mental hygiene law with the following responsibilities, among others: "to conduct studies into the causes, nature and treatment of diseases affecting the mind, brain and nervous system; to discover and apply more efficient measures of prevention, treatment and cure of such disorders in order that their numbers shall be decreased; and to develop methods of prevention and cure through an out-patient department." The research interests and activities of the Psychiatric Institute and its associated institutions have been described in the earlier report on research in state hospitals and other tax-supported institutions for the mentally ill and defective.

In addition, the department engages in extensive researches of a statistical nature which are carried on by the Bureau of Statistics at the central office in Albany. The bureau regularly collects statistics on many and varied aspects of the operations of the state institutions, and its annual compilations provide a vast amount of source material for its researches and studies, which contribute basically to the clinical researches of the institutions. Its productiveness is attested by numerous original studies and analyses that have enriched the scientific literature in

101

this field over a period of years. Outstanding among its recent contributions have been its study of hereditary and environmental factors in the causation of dementia praecox and the manic-depressive psychoses; a study of the social and biological aspects of mental disease based on statistical analyses of case records showing the relation of mental disease to age, sex, environment, marriage, nativity and race; studies of the efficacy of insulin and metrazol shock therapies; and various studies dealing with expectation and outcome of mental disease, and its social and economic significance.

Current researches include an evaluation of results obtained by electric shock therapy; racial distribution of admissions to state schools for mental defectives; and studies of parole and family care conducted jointly by selected state hospitals and the Temporary Commission on State Hospital Problems. The department is also engaged in the preparation of "A Comprehensive History of the Care of the Insane in the State of New York." Until the summer of 1942 this project was carried on with the aid of personnel from the Federal Works Progress Administration under the supervision of the Bureau of Statistics.

BALTIMORE, MD.

The Children's Rehabilitation Institute

This is a private voluntary school and training center accommodating some 50 children of all ages who are afflicted with cerebral palsy but are of the higher grades of intelligence (above the level of mental deficiency). It has a regular consulting psychiatrist who is also on the faculty of psychiatry at Johns Hopkins. While its work is primarily concerned with physiotherapy, occupational therapy and education, it gives a great deal of attention to the adjustment problems of its children and has accumulated an experience and a file of case records that are unusual in this respect. In addition, it encounters many psychologic adjustment problems in the child-parent relationship. Its interest in the behavior problems of the child looks, in one direction, to the attitudes of the parent toward the child, especially in the matter of overprotection, and in another, toward the non-psychological determinants of conduct disorders.

BOSTON, MASS.

Massachusetts Department of Mental Health

Aside from the researches conducted in the individual state institutions, the staff of the central office of the Massachusetts Department of Mental Health is itself active in research, in two directions: statistics and administration.

The statistical research is based upon a punch card system whereby every new patient admitted to a hospital is represented by a statistical card in the department's files. Each time a change occurs in the status of the patient, a new statistical entry is made—as when on visit, on discharge or readmission. The readmission card is cumulative—superseding all previous cards. With these data and the use of mechanical classification, large numbers of correlations can be achieved.

These have already resulted in outstanding reports of a statistical nature which give leads for clinical research in the individual hospitals. Statistical analysis of the records of individual hospital patients provides similar leads for research. Thus, the department is in a position to assist the various institutions in selecting patients for specific research projects. For instance, if a hospital wishes to know the names of patients diagnosed "catatonic dementia praecox," say between the ages of 20 and 40, the department can furnish the requested data in a day or two. It also serves individual workers who wish help in organizing researches, by guiding and assisting them to set up their codes, determine criteria, punch the cards, draw up tables, etc. In some instances this may involve two or three months of work by department personnel.

A notable example of statistical research achieved on the basis of the department's system of recording and reporting mental diseases is the comprehensive study of statistical trends conducted by the department during 1928–1939—one of the most extensive projects ever undertaken by statisticians in this field. This study, which analyzes the sociological, clinical and other factors in the histories of 89,190 patients admitted or readmitted to all mental hospitals in the State of Massachusetts over a 17-year period, from 1917 to 1933, gives a broad and illuminating picture of the widespread incidence and social significance of mental disorders that will be of great value to students of this important public health problem for years to come. (See "New Facts on Mental Disorders," by Neil Dayton. 1940. Chas. C. Thomas, Springfield, Ill.)

The administrative research of the department is based on the principle that administrative mishaps—suicide, escape, injury, etc.—are not mere matters of chance. By combined analyses of such mishaps by the hospital personnel, the contributory and causative factors are isolated and preventive measures are evolved. The procedure followed is to deal with these matters, as one does in clinical investigations, as symptoms to be understood and managed.

Supreme Council, 33°, Scottish Rite, Northern Masonic Jurisdiction, U. S. A.

This fraternal organization has adopted the support of research into dementia praecox as its major benevolence and is devoting some $45,000 a year to investigations in this field. It operates through The National Committee for Mental Hygiene, which administers the program under the direction of an advisory committee composed of outstanding representatives of psychiatry and allied medical sciences. Dr. Nolan D. C. Lewis, Director of the New York State Psychiatric Institute and Hospital, is field representative and coördinator of the program. Most of the grants are made to hospitals and universities discussed in other parts of this report. Some 70 investigators in 14 scientific centers have been engaged on 30 or more research problems during the past seven years in what is a coördinated, long-range study of the disorder in its various ramifications. Workers in psychiatry, neurology, psychology, physiology, chemistry, genetics, and other biological disciplines, have united their efforts in a comprehensive and integrated attack on fundamental aspects of this many-sided problem. Subsidies have been made for the year 1941–42 to the following investigators who with their associates are working on projects within their special spheres of scientific interest and study:

Dr. John C. Whitehorn, Phipps Psychiatric Clinic, Baltimore, Md.

Dr. Charles Bradley, Emma Pendleton Bradley Home, East Providence, R. I.

Dr. Margarethe A. Ribble, New York, N. Y.

Dr. Heinrich Klüver, University of Chicago, Chicago, Ill.

Dr. Solomon Katzenelbogen, St. Elizabeths Hospital, Washington, D. C.

Dr. Detlev W. Bronk, University of Pennsylvania, Philadelphia, Pa.

Dr. Carl F. Schmidt, University of Pennsylvania, Philadelphia, Pa.

Dr. Joseph Hughes, Institute of the Pennsylvania Hospital, Philadelphia, Pa.

Dr. Nolan D. C. Lewis, New York State Psychiatric Institute, New York, N. Y.

Dr. Esther Bogen Tietz (formerly Longview Hospital, Cincinnati, Ohio).

Dr. Margaret Mead, American Museum of Natural History, New York, N. Y.

Dr. J. D. M. Griffin and Dr. William Line, University of Toronto, Toronto, Canada.

Dr. George H. Bishop, Washington University, St. Louis, Mo.

Dr. William G. Lennox, Boston City Hospital, Boston, Mass.

Dr. Lauretta Bender, Bellevue Psychiatric Hospital, New York, N. Y.

Mrs. Lois Paul, Chicago, Ill.

H. Edmund Bullis, Delaware Society for Mental Hygiene, Wilmington, Del.

Dr. Reginald Lourie, New York, N. Y.

The investigations cover a wide range of problems, involving observation, study and experimentation in the realms of ethnology, heredity, infant growth and behavior, biochemistry, neurophysics, clinical pathology and psychiatry, education and sociology. Clinical studies include an evaluation and comparative study of schizophrenic patients responding to insulin treatment, and inquiries into the nature of "schizophrenic thinking"; evaluation of the effects of drug therapies on conduct disorders in children, and follow-up studies of children previously treated whose behavior was thought to be characteristic of schizophrenia; behavior problems of early infancy and their relations to later development of mental disorders; the relation of extreme shyness and timidity in school children to subsequent dementia-praecox symptoms; and a study of maturation and function of the autonomic nervous system in children with dementia praecox.

Laboratory studies deal with mechanisms involved in eidetic imagery and other sensory deceptions, a study of hallucinations and other behavior changes experimentally produced by mescaline and related chemical substances, analysis of functions of the temporal lobes, and anatomical changes secondary to temporal lobectomy; studies in neurophysics, including the effects of drugs and chemicals on synaptic connections and on nerve conduction, experimental techniques for determination of oxygen exchange in tissues and oxygen tension in intercellular fluids of the brain, and neurophysiology of the spinal cord; quantitative measurement of cerebral blood flow; influence of chemical agents on nerve excitation and inhibition in the respiratory center in the brains of experimental animals; the effects of pharmacological, electric shock and fever therapies on adrenalin balance in the blood; analysis of stimulation and responses of the optic nerve and related investigations of the brain cortex; and electroencephalographic studies in the differentiation of brain waves and their sources.

Studies of constitution and heredity have been pointed toward the relation of body development, inheritance and growth factors to dementia praecox and other personality disorders; the specificity and manifestations of predisposition to schizophrenia, and the genetic relationship between the tendency to schizophrenia and hereditary low resistance to tuberculosis as evidenced by statistical and clinical studies of several hundred pairs of twins.

Ethnological investigations include studies conducted by an anthropologist among the aboriginal tribes of Bali, in which parent-child behavior, symbolic play, trance phenomena, social sanctions and other aspects of Balinese culture have been observed for factors suggestice of schizoid personality characteristics; and an anthropological study of primitive children in San Pedro, Guatemala, which is concerned with the anxieties, hostilities and family relationships of these children and the way they are expressed in a situation where there is a fairly constant cultural norm.

CHICAGO, ILL.

Institute of General Semantics

The Institute of General Semantics is a non-profit school for the promulgation of the principles of general semantics and for experimentation in their application to problems of human evaluating reactions. Its director is the outstanding contributor to and interpreter of this field, and has associated with him men from other nearby and distant institutions. The empirical work of this school attempts to test and study the application of the principles of general semantics to non-psychotic persons as a process of mental hygiene. This process is directed particularly to persons whose problems are within the range of the rational approach. Its subjects are professional students in the school who are given instruction and who are observed for related changes in behavior. Many reports are issued by the Institute and there is a growing literature on semantics inspired by the activities of this center.

DETROIT, MICH.

Henry Ford Hospital

The Henry Ford Hospital is a voluntary general hospital designed to receive its support from those benefiting from its services. Its neuropsychiatric service is deliberately distributed among the other services of the hospital, thereby breaking down all isolation of the field and insuring the advantages of neuropsychiatric procedures to all patients to whom they may apply. This also necessitates the provision of adequate nursing and other facilities in order to avoid mechanical, chemical or other doubtful shortcuts to the management of administratively difficult symptoms. The division of neuropsychiatry is thus, in its whole set-up, experimental in character and conduct and at the same time designed to contribute in a practical way to the maintenance of high standards of care and treatment. Only the most violent or noisy patients cannot be handled in this way, but this type of patient is admitted, is treated in intensive manner, and often during his convalescence is transferred to other floors in the hospital.

While all types of neuropsychiatric cases are admitted, the program is especially adapted to the treatment of psychoneurotic patients, who comprise the greatest number of in-patients, and these are given continuous study. The traumatic neuroses are of special interest. Similarly a critical study of sedatives and analgesics has been included in the investigative activities. An endeavor is under way to develop substitutes for opiates in conjunction with surgical treatment. Epidurography is another line of special interest. Some attention is given to the relation between body-type glandular functions and mental characteristics, and one member of the staff is studying the parent-child relationship in cases of illegitimacy. Aside from these trends, incidental studies are undertaken from time to time as provocative clinical material appears on the service.

The hospital accommodates from 25 to 60 neuropsychiatric in-patients on eight or more different floors. The staff includes four psychiatrists, two neurologists, two psychologists, one resident psychiatrist and one resident neurologist. The neuropsychiatric service includes many consultations with other divisions of the hospital and an out-patient department. The hospital has excellent library facilities, including the important psychiatric periodical literature. The laboratories are mostly clinical adjuncts, but foster research liberally. Occasional neuropathological collaboration is secured from Wayne University. While research is not a primary objective of the hospital, investigation is encouraged as an expression of individual interest and initiative.

KANSAS CITY, MO.

Neurological Hospital

This is a proprietary mental hospital with a capacity of 49 beds and an average daily population of 29 patients. During 1940 there were 160 first admissions, of which the great majority were psychoses of various types. There is a staff of three full-time psychiatrists, a neurologist and neurosurgeon, with a complement of three graduate nurses and 13 attendants, and a part-time laboratory technician. A department of neurosurgery and neurology was recently established to provide better integration of psychiatric and neurologic work. There are no residents or internes, but medical students are occasionally employed in the laboratory or on the wards. One member of the staff is consultant to the Kansas City General Hospital; another is on·the active staff of the Kansas City General Hospital and on the faculty of the University of Kansas School of Medicine. The latter also holds an appointment as special lecturer in neurology and psychiatry at the Kansas City Western Dental College and lectures on psychiatry at several schools of nursing.

There is a library of 500 medical books and several journals, including some dealing with various medical specialties. The laboratory is equipped to do routine work and other facilities in the city are available for autopsies, serological and tissue work. There is also apparatus for encephalographic work and electric shock therapy.

The major research interests of the institution at the present time are in three fields, namely, the psychiatry of old age, nutritional deficiencies in major psychoses, and insulin treatment of delirium tremens. Reports have been published on work in progress, including several papers on shock therapy in patients over 35 years of age, and several on the effects of drugs in the treatment of alcoholism. The emphasis in research at this center at the present time is shifting toward a study of the various psychotic manifestations seen in the older patients. A series of reports correlating findings and observations in the toxic delirious reactions of old age are now in preparation.

KATONAH, N. Y.

Pinewood

This modestly conducted proprietary mental hospital of some 50 beds has a distinctly inquiring spirit. It is equipped with a laboratory designed for the usual clinical needs, but has access to the Northern Westchester Hospital for roentgenological work and to the Neurological

Institute in New York City for other special laboratory work. It is related by appointment of staff members to Vanderbilt Clinic, Neurological Institute, Yonkers General Hospital, and Hillside Hospital (formerly Hastings Hillside Hospital). The library of the hospital contains all the important psychiatric and neurological periodicals and, in addition, there is access to the library of the Academy of Medicine in New York City.

Research and experimentation have been directed toward studies in shock therapy; Pinewood was among the first institutions to utilize insulin shock treatment in America. Metrazol and electric convulsive treatments were also used at Pinewood from their incipiency. Studies of the technique and complications of metrazol and electric shock treatment were recently completed. Pinewood has also engaged in research on the problem of addictions, particularly alcohol. Reports of this institution's researches appear in the scientific literature from time to time.

NEW YORK, N. Y.

Committee for the Study of Sex Variants

The Committee for the Study of Sex Variants differs from other centers included in this report in that it is not a physical set-up, but an organization for the coördination and stimulation of research that is carried on through individual efforts. It has no laboratory, library or clinical facilities or formal patients of its own.

The Committee's study covers potentially all types of sex variant and many of these have already come within its scope. The main attention has been directed toward a study of some 80 male and female homosexuals of a more intelligent class who have been privately referred for psychiatric study. Much time and effort, at their own expense, has been devoted by those participating in the study.

In addition to exhaustive life studies, including as much as possible of pertinent data obtained by interview, physi-

cal examinations, biochemical, roentgenological and photographic procedures, and special psychological tests of
masculinity-femininity, have been made, and the New York
Hospital has assisted in these in an informal way.

All this provides a wealth of source material which was
recently published in two volumes. The report presents
the individual studies in detail and also the cumulative
studies cutting across the 80 cases.

Hillside Hospital, Queens, N. Y.

Research at this hospital, formerly known as Hastings
Hillside Hospital and located at Hastings-on-Hudson, New
York, is very much the expression of the interests of its
director. The hospital is a voluntary institution accommodating about 80 mental patients. A new hospital was
recently constructed in Queens Borough, New York City,
where provision is being made for laboratories and an
expanded library. The former will be equipped for biochemical and psychological studies. The present library
collection includes the important neurological and psychiatric periodicals and reprints. The staff includes five full-
time psychiatrists and one half-time assistant.

The research interests of this hospital tend toward
studies of constitution. A study has been started of estrogenic substances in the various functional psychoses, and
electrocardiographic studies have been made of patients
under treatment with metrazol and continued with patients
under electric shock therapy. Clinical experimentation with
group psychotherapy and group interaction of patients has
been in progress for some time. The hospital has an
organization of its former patients 'through whom it
attempts to improve the popular attitude toward mental
hospitals and to reduce resistance to early treatment of
mental disease.

The Jewish Board of Guardians

The Jewish Board of Guardians is a quasi-psychiatric
agency which provides social case work and limited psy-

chiatric service to non-institutional children with behavior problems in New York City, and to two institutions for boys and girls, respectively, at Hawthorne and Cedar Knolls, N. Y. For the former it has a staff of part-time psychiatrists equivalent to nearly two persons on full time, one psychologist, 46 staff case workers, and some 10 students from Smith College and the New York School of Social Work. A part of the requirement for a degree for these students is a thesis. While such theses often represent a creditable piece of original scientific work dependent upon clinical research and experimentation, and are carefully planned and supervised, they express no special trend of investigation. The institutional aspect of the agency's function is covered by a staff of one full-time and one half-time psychiatrist, one half-time psychologist, and six social workers. The agency has a small scientific library at headquarters, including books and some 17 of the more pertinent scientific periodicals.

Financial provision for research is not a part of the regular budget, but it is supported by special grants. Research is largely an expression of individual interest, but the accumulation of records of children with behavior problems and the current service to such children turns the investigations in the direction of follow-up and clinical studies. One study deals with a five-year follow-up of 465 boys formerly at Hawthorne, to determine their present status in relation to initial diagnosis and subsequent method of treatment. Another follow-up evaluates the effects of child guidance treatment on individual behavior over a selected period of years.

The Lifwynn Foundation

The work of The Lifwynn Foundation consists essentially of the personal efforts of a small group of psychiatrists and their associates, held together by a common orientation and served by a common laboratory. They are interested in bringing to bear upon the function of man as a species the findings of psychiatric experience with inter-individual imbalances in human relations, together with the results of experimental studies in human motivation designed to enrich, test and elucidate clinical experience. It is aimed thereby to rid the functioning of man (culture, international relations, etc.) of the unconscious forces that reduce his biological and social effectiveness. These forces are frequently evidenced by muscular, respiratory, ocular and other tensions, certain new effects of which have already been reported by the Foundation and are subject to further study by special apparatus for observing and recording such tensions.

In addition to this equipment in its own laboratories, working relations exist with laboratories at Harvard University, Cornell University Medical School, Fordham University, University of Chicago, New York University, Presbyterian Hospital and Brooklyn Jewish Hospital, where other special tests and apparatus are obtained as needed. Several commercial firms have also coöperated in supplying drugs or technical help. These outside sources greatly extend the potentialities for research in the Foundation's laboratories.

The scientific staff consists of three psychiatrists, a psychologist, and a laboratory director who hold appointments also at the New York Hospital and Cornell University Medical School, at Bellevue Hospital and the New York University Medical School. The library includes standard reference books in medicine, biology and related sciences, and the more important general medical, psychiatric and psychological periodicals, both domestic and foreign.

While there is an endowment, this is not large enough to provide for anything but accessories. The Foundation's income consists largely of contributions from its scientific staff and its few working members. The time of the staff is in large part volunteered, but the research projects are seriously handicapped by a lack of funds. The members of the scientific staff not only conduct the research, but by the very nature of their undertaking they serve as subjects upon whom the investigations are carried out. The research projects reported from time to time amply testify to the productive activity of the organization.

Mt. Sinai Hospital

Mt. Sinai Hospital is a voluntary general hospital with a psychiatric service both for the wards and for the out-patient department. This psychiatric service is an administrative subdivision of the neurological department. The psychiatric in-patients are preponderantly patients of the medical, surgical and specialty services, and of the neurological wards as well. A few patients with neurotic disturbances are admitted directly to the neurological wards for special study; but there are no special beds for psychiatric patients as such. The out-patient clinic admits no patients directly from the outside, but serves the other departments in the out-patient department, and secondarily, patients discharged from the wards with neurotic disturbances. There is a daily morning out-patient clinic attended by about 30 visiting psychiatrists, each serving three days a week. Other psychiatrists are assigned to duty as "roving psychiatrists" to take consultations in other clinics of the out-patient department. Furthermore, smaller groups of psychiatrists are attached permanently to other clinics, such as the medical clinics, the menopause clinic, gastroenterology, etc. Finally there is a special division of the psychiatric clinic for the care of the more chronic neuroses. The psychiatrists assigned to the wards are organized into sub-units of two or three psychiatrists, each such unit being attached to a special service.

The laboratories of the hospital are designed for the most part for clinical service, and have been productive centers of investigation for years. Particularly is this true of the neuropathology laboratory. The hospital has an excellent medical library, but is so close to the New York Academy of Medicine that the library of the latter is extensively used.

The very nature of the hospital, and the form of its

organization with a staff of psychiatrists who are largely engaged in private practice, fits in with a major interest in psychosomatic problems. Special attention is given to the psychiatric orientation of the house staff and the younger attending physicians of all of the other services.

Problems that are receiving special attention at the present time include colitis, hypertension, coronary disease, skin allergies, thyroid disorders, menopausal problems, emotional disturbances in reaction to surgery, postoperative delirium, etc. Special electroencephalographic equipment is available and is used in studying the effects of forms of slow medication, especially of sedatives. Induced communicative sleep is under investigation. Other studies include special problems in the pharmacology of anxiety states, and personality problems of epileptic children.

While there are no formal affiliations between Mt. Sinai Hospital and other research centers in the city, and while the staff members have appointments at many other hospitals, and all the medical schools, the relation to Columbia Medical Center is functionally the closest.

Another aspect of psychiatric service at Mt. Sinai Hospital is that rendered by the pediatric department, especially through the out-patient Children's Health Class, although ward patients in the children's department are also seen upon request. The pediatric department has its own organization in the form of a regular child guidance clinic, with three psychiatrically trained pediatricians in attendance, a full-time psychologist, and three psychiatric social workers. It also maintains a speech department for the remedial correction of speech defects in children under the care of the department.

The Children's Health Class is concerned with the various problems of children, in terms of emotional, educational and social maladjustment, and the care and treatment of neurotics and incipient psychotics, as well as the prevention of delinquency. All of the hospital's facilities are utilized in the research activities of this department, which have been developed particularly along psychological and social lines.   The problems receiving main study at the Children's Health Class at the present time include the relations of graphology, palmistry and the Rorschach test, the study of precocious puberty, studies of capillaries in problem children, and some analyses of the constancy of the intelligence quotient and reasons for its deviation.

New York Infirmary for Women and Children

The New York Infirmary for Women and Children is, as its name implies, not specifically a psychiatric institution. It is in position, however, to foster the study of children, from birth through adolescence, and of the child-parent relationship, beginning in the prenatal period. For some years it has had a staff consultant whose time has been devoted to research into the relation of development and growth—physiological, constitutional, congenital, and psychobiological—to inter-personal and situational experiences.   It is concerned with the effect of such experiences on physiological function as well as the reverse.

The research subjects consist of 47 children and their parents and, in a few cases, siblings who for the past 13 years or so (beginning at the age of 6 weeks) have been studied periodically from many different angles. In addition, 10 cases have been studied from the prenatal period on, though some, of course, have been lost. Each study (treatment inevitably goes along with study) has been both pediatric and psychiatric. The emphasis in research approach has been on the practical application of the knowledge gained from the various studies to clinical work with children and parents, and for purposes of prevention. The broad scope of these studies is reflected, among other things, in their follow-through from infancy to the pre-adolescent and adolescent periods and, especially, their concern with the relationship of adolescence to early childhood. Special techniques of examining behavior in infants and children have been used and adapted. Psychometric studies of both intelligence and achievement are a part of the follow-up procedure. All of the resources of the hospital—laboratory, library, bed and out-patient services and social services—are available, as well as the special quarters assigned to the consultant for these studies.

Outside contacts afford opportunities to test, in practice, the findings and results of these studies. The consultant is an assistant lecturer at New York University Medical College. She has an informal arrangement for the exchange of reports with school-teachers of the children studied, and similar contacts with camps and settlements to which the children and their parents may go. Findings are also tested out through preparatory education of parents for delivery and psychiatric study during and after pregnancy; through prognoses as to development each year, with rechecking; through consultation service to an agency concerned with adoption; and through anthropological field studies. Studies of the effects of different frustrations on infants and children are in progress. The extensive records used in these researches include motion pictures, stills and special charts, as well as the usual written reports. An effort is under way to apply the findings in the various studies to the work of maternal and child health centers and through coöperation between the Department of Health and the Board of Education. The material also provided a basis for a suggested national program of health-education which was prepared by this center for consideration by the United States Public Health Service in 1937, and was later revised for the fostering of morale as well as health during the emergency. A number of scientific articles emanating from these studies have already been published.

The New York Vocational Adjustment Bureau for Girls*

While not specifically a psychiatric agency, the Vocational Adjustment Bureau includes in its work studies that

* See footnote, page 162.

are psychiatrically important in their implications or that are specifically psychiatric in their processes. It is a privately supported philanthropic agency founded by Mrs. Henry Ittleson in 1919, and specializing in the study of problem girls, particularly in relation to vocational guidance and employment. The social, educational and physical history of each individual is considered. The Bureau's objective is to determine scientifically the potential abilities of its clients, emphasizing the mental efficiency factor particularly as it applies to the schizoid and manic personalities. The studies reveal the special abilities of the low grade group and the weaknesses of those of superior intelligence.

The Bureau maintains its offices in a large vocational high school for girls and serves practically all of the social agencies, and many of the clinics, hospitals, and schools in and about New York City. It offers facilities, too, for the testing and study of girls and women paroled from state hospitals and correctional institutions. The Bureau is always actively engaged in practical research studies that may throw light upon increasing the productivity and happy adjustment of members of this group. In 1937–39 an experiment to determine the possibilities of mental hygiene service at the kindergarten level was carried on by a complete psychiatric clinical unit in coöperation with the New York Board of Education.

In coöperation with the Board of Education the Bureau has carried on special unit training courses to prepare for employment girls in the lower intelligence brackets. For more than 10 years a "Sheltered Workshop" was conducted on a commercial basis, where the mentally handicapped functioned productively under supervision. The agency also serves as a training center for students from Columbia University and the College of the City of New York, who receive credit for internships that may lead to advanced degrees.

OSSINING, N. Y.

Stony Lodge

Stony Lodge is a proprietary mental hospital of some 30 patients for whom there is a staff of five psychiatrists. The entire staff participates directly or indirectly in research activities and has been recognized for years as a contributor to the scientific literature. Its laboratory facilities are designed primarily as clinical adjuncts. Its library has all the psychiatric and the more important psychological and social periodicals, and there is access to the libraries of the New York State Psychiatric Institute, the New York Hospital, and the Academy of Medicine for more extensive references. Members of the staff have affiliations with Vanderbilt Clinic and the College of Physicians and Surgeons at the Columbia Medical Center, and Lenox Hill Hospital. Researches are directed especially toward clinical chemotherapeutic investigation. It has pioneered in experimentation with the several shock therapies. It is at present engaged in a study of the reaction of patients to acetylcholine. This is conducted jointly with the Department of Psychiatry of Columbia University. A research project in group psychotherapy is also in progress. In prospect is a clinical study of obsessive compulsion psychoneuroses from records of former patients.

PROVIDENCE, R. I.

Butler Hospital
Emma Pendleton Bradley Home

Psychiatric research in Providence emanates primarily from two centers: Butler Hospital and the Emma Pendleton Bradley Home. Closely related to each other, as they have been, under a common management, over a period of 10 years, their close-knit relations with many medical, health and welfare services of the community afford a much broader investigative resource than these institutions would provide by themselves.

Bradley Home is a 50-bed hospital for children with neurological and psychiatric disorders, one of the very few institutions of its type in this country. Its professional personnel includes a resident physician, two interns of pediatric background, psychologists, eight' psychological interns, school-teachers, a recreational director, and a biochemist, in addition to nursing staff. Nursery as well as grade school facilities are provided. Some members of the staff have outside connections. The teaching of abnormal psychology and psychometrics (as applied to children) is carried on for Brown University by staff members who utilize the excellent resources of Bradley Home for this purpose. Graduate students occasionally conduct studies here in fulfillment of requirements for advanced degrees. Lectures are given to nurses on child psychiatry and post-graduate training is also offered for nurses in this field. The training program for resident psychiatrists of Butler Hospital and the Rhode Island State Hospital includes an elective three-months' period at Bradley Home, and special trainees in pediatrics at Tufts College Medical School likewise spend some time here.

The institution has laboratory facilities for biochemical, psychological and electroencephalographic studies adequate for current projects, but capable of expansion as needed. Its library includes the more important psychiatric and pediatric journals and provision is made for the regular purchase of new books. The resources of the Boston Medical Library are available through the library of the Rhode Island Medical Society. The Psychological Library at Brown University is available too.

The researches of Bradley Home include a monographic study of early schizophrenia, pharmacological treatment of conduct disorders, and study of convulsive disorders and behavior problems as influenced by drugs and reflected by electroencephalographic changes. A concurrent attempt is under way to establish electroencephalographic norms.

Follow up studies have been undertaken on children diagnosed as schizophrenic or schizoid who have been under observation in and out of the hospital for periods ranging from four to nine years. Also in progress is some intensive investigation of the effect of curare on children with cerebral palsy.

Biochemical studies include the development of quantitative methods for acetone and B-oxybutyric acid in blood and urine. Some psychosomatic studies have also been made. Research by all staff members is encouraged. Each year two psychological interns are taken on who conduct the routine testing at the hospital and who, during their year's internship, are expected to complete some research project appropriate to their background and special interests.

Butler Hospital is a long-established voluntary institution, with a capacity of some 170 beds for all types of patients and a staff including 11 psychiatrists. Its ties with Providence and Rhode Island generally bring it into close touch with all aspects of human welfare locally and it serves as a hospital for state patients in addition to the Rhode Island State Hospital. It also has ties of an informal sort with the state hospital in the training of young physicians in psychiatry, and in exchanging the attendance of personnel at staff conferences. In addition, the superintendent is advisor to the State Welfare Advisory Council, and an officer of the Emma Pendleton Bradley Home, at East Providence. Several staff members hold teaching appointments at Brown University and use the hospital's resources for teaching purposes. Other appointments include Rhode Island Hospital, Lying-In Hospital, Pawtucket Memorial Hospital, Charles V. Chapin Hospital, Homeopathic Hospital, Bradley Home, Providence Child Guidance Clinic, Yale University, and local welfare agencies, including the Community Chest, Council of Social Agencies, Visiting Nurse Association, and Neighborhood Bureau. Students from 14 nursing schools receive affiliate psychiatric training here.

Butler Hospital has an up-to-date medical library, with a full-time and a part-time librarian, and including the important psychiatric journals. Regular staff conferences are held for the review of literature. Psychological, electroencephalographic, and clinical laboratory facilities are available, sufficient for present researches. The researches are primarily clinical, although some are primarily investigative. The staff includes a full-time psychologist who is studying psychological (memory) changes incident to shock treatment, by serial testing of patients. In a study of language development in the individual a conditioning technique is employed. Schizophrenic patients are studied to determine metabolic and respiratory changes under emotional stimuli, and associative processes. Organic brain changes are considered through the study of verbal and judgmental changes observed in frontal lobectomy and Rorschach characteristics of organic aphasias. Pick's disease is being studied by psychological tests and tests of localization.

RICHMOND, VA.

Tucker Hospital

This proprietary neuropsychiatric hospital of 50 beds and three physicians located in the heart of Richmond, Va., is related functionally to many other centers of psychiatric activity. Its chief of staff is on the board of the Nemours Foundation, which conducts an institution for handicapped children, and in which mental considerations are given a large place. A process of observing behavior in well children is now being developed. All members of the staff hold appointments at the Medical College of Virginia and serve in its hospital division, and one is psychiatrist to the state prison. One is associated with the American Hospital in Paris, under whose ægis studies have been pursued abroad. Two hold appointments at the local Hospital for Crippled Children and one is on the executive board of the local Child Guidance Clinic.

The laboratories of this hospital are developed for clinical routine tests, and other laboratories in the city are used for special purposes, including neuropsychology. The library is equipped with standard books and the leading psychiatric and neurological periodicals.

Researches include both clinical and basic investigations. The hypothalamus has been the subject of special attention under a foundation grant. Several reports have already been issued. Clinical investigations have centered on neurological and psychiatric concomitants of albinism, neuropathological studies of shock treatment, yeast meningitis, heredity of myopathic disorders, and critical evaluation of fever therapy in neuropsychiatry.

Westbrook Sanitarium

This proprietary mental hospital situated in the environs of Richmond, Va., accommodates 130 patients, and has a staff of six physicians. Its research output varies and is largely dependent upon individual initiative. The investigations are clinical in nature. The laboratory facilities are designed for clinical routine tests. The library includes the outstanding neurological, psychiatric and general medical periodicals, as well as standard books. Clinical studies directed toward therapy include modifications of shock therapy, use of codein in the treatment of morphinism and of sodium chloride in delirium tremens; and those concerned with diagnosis include correlations of blood, alcohol and behavior variations in hypoglycemia in mental maladjustment, symptomatic significance of achlorhydria, and correlation of alcoholism and pellagra.

ROCKVILLE, MD.

Chestnut Lodge Sanitarium

This proprietary mental hospital has a capacity of 45 beds and a staff of 10 psychiatrists, four of whom are qualified psychoanalysts. In its research it functions independently of other institutions. In the past two years it has contributed some excellent articles to the scientific literature. Laboratory facilities are limited to the needs of regular clinical work and library facilities chiefly to psychiatric and psychoanalytic periodicals. The rich library resources of nearby Washington are also available.

The research interests of this institution are distinctly psychoanalytic and are directed toward the development of psychoanalytically oriented treatment of the psychoses, a field that has not been extensively developed by psychoanalysts. Current investigations include studies of the effects of analysis on patients, the effects of patients undergoing analysis on other patients, and the relationship between patients, staff and other personnel with special reference to discernible trends influencing both individuals and groups.

SAN FRANCISCO, CAL.

Mount Zion Hospital

Mount Zion Hospital is a voluntary general hospital, supported in part by the Community Chest of San Francisco, and contributing substantially to the mental health needs of the community. Its psychiatric service functions as part of the out-patient department and is staffed by two full-time psychiatrists, one half-time psychiatrist, two volunteer part-time psychiatrists, one full-time social worker, two students in training, and one part-time volunteer psychologist. Its social service facilities are supplemented by case-work services rendered by the Jewish Family Service Agency. There are no hospital beds devoted exclusively to psychiatric patients, but milder cases are admitted to the general wards, and provisions have been made for electric shock therapy and psychiatric observation. Eligibility for treatment in the out-patient department has been liberally interpreted, with the result that the psychiatric division has been able to render a wider community service than other departments of the hospital.

The psychiatric service is engaging in several research projects, mostly of a clinical nature. Among these is a study of psychodynamic factors in schizophrenia; a study of personality changes following substitution therapy in pre-adolescent eunuchoidism; an experiment in group treatment of neurotic adolescent girls; and a study of the factors that enter into the success or failure of foster home and institutional placement of children.

STOCKBRIDGE, MASS.

Austen Riggs Foundation, Inc.

The Austen Riggs Foundation, Inc., is a non-profit-making, therapeutic center for the care and treatment of patients suffering from disorders of a psychoneurotic nature. It provides housing facilities for a maximum of 50 patients and operates an occupational therapy department. It supplies funds to a certain number of patients unable to pay the regular charges for treatment and maintenance. The teaching of graduate physicians has always been an essential part of its function.

The professional staff consists of a group of psychiatrists practicing under the name of the Austen Riggs Associates. An office in New York is maintained which offers both a pre- and post-treatment consultation service to patients. The Foundation supports a clinic in Pittsfield, Mass., and provides a consultation service for Vassar and Williams Colleges and the House of Mercy Hospital in Pittsfield, Mass.

While the Foundation has adjunct laboratory service as needed for its clinical work and has access to nearby laboratory resources where needed, its research interests and opportunities are mainly of a clinical and therapeutic nature. It has library facilities, including some 25 of the most important psychiatric and medical periodicals.

Research is an integral part of its function. A report embodying the findings of four years of research into the psychoneuroses, sponsored by the Markle Foundation, has recently been published. Currently a survey is being made of psychiatric services offered by the New England colleges. This is being financed by former patients.

TOPEKA, KANS.

Menninger Sanitarium and Clinic and Southard School

These institutions form the only active research center in Topeka. The Menninger Sanitarium is a private corporation staffed by the psychiatrists, physicians, neurologists and psychologists of the Menninger Clinic and serving those suffering from functional and organic diseases of the nervous system, in both residential and out-patient services. Other functions include counsel in child guidance, industrial psychiatry, marital relations, and a consultation service to outside physicians in local hospitals. The Southard School, designed for children with problems of adjustment—not mental deficiency—is a voluntary (nonprofit) institution for research, teaching and treatment. The staffs of the sanitarium, clinic and school are intimately linked, the sanitarium having a capacity of 60 in-patients, the school 20. The group issues a bimonthly periodical, the *Bulletin of the Menninger Clinic*, in which the results of researches, chiefly of this group, are reported. The evidences of research productivity are abundant in the psychiatric literature, the size and variety of the staff and the highly developed, and in some respects unique, clinical resources of this center making possible a wide scope of research interests. Much effort has gone into the development of new and improved diagnostic, therapeutic and educational techniques and devices and their application to resident patients, both at the clinic and the school.

There is also an extensive resident training program, with considerable experimental activity in psychiatric education for various professional groups, as well as a working relationship with outside groups and institutions. The psychoanalysts on the staff form the nucleus of the

Topeka Psychoanalytic Society, which is the branch of the American Psychoanalytic Association functioning for the western half of the United States. They are also closely related in a teaching and consultative capacity to the local Washburn Municipal University, and staff members are also on the faculties of the University of Kansas and Washington University, St. Louis (Kansas City Branch).

Educational experimentation at the center includes preparation of psychiatric data for group presentation, for psychiatric training purposes, to nurses, doctors, psychiatric residents and psychological interns, and the application of psychiatry to education, industry, military training, social work and the personal problems of college students. Institutes are held annually for school teachers, pediatricians, and psychiatrists on problems of adult-child relationships. Experimentation is also directed toward hospital administrative problems, particularly the development of greater specificity in the use of treatment devices and the development of more precise theory and direction for occupational therapy.

While there is a distinct psychoanalytic orientation in this center, its investigations cover a broad range of problems, of both laboratory and clinical character. Adjunct facilities for research include neuropathological, psychological, X-ray and chemistry laboratories, and pneumo- and electroencephalographic apparatus for diagnostic research. Investigative activities include a study of the pharmacodynamics and psychological effects of metrazol and its therapeutic use in barbiturate intoxication. Detailed psychological studies of metrazol and electric shock and other therapeutic procedures represent another line of interest. Attention is given to such specific questions as mycropsia, relation of ordinal position of siblings to choice of profession, twinship, color response, character formation and frustration in psychiatric patients. Other psychiatric projects deal with psychosomatic problems, such as asthma, peptic ulcer, and hypertension, with follow-up studies of influenza, emotional reactions to physical examinations, and studies of personality structure in normal individuals. Special attention is given to suicide, particularly the function of woman in our culture in relation to suicide.

The application of psychoanalysis and special psychotherapies to institutional cases, and in relation to short-term treatment, provide another point of departure for research activity. Psychoanalytic studies of alcohol and drug addiction are reinforced by special Rorschach and other psychological studies. Modified psychoanalytic techniques are used in treating psychotic patients, and psychoanalytic principles are applied to mental hygiene consultation and short-term psychotherapy. Special attention is given to anxiety, traumatic neurosis and emotions in speech and language difficulties, and a critical survey is being made of treatment procedures in schizophrenia, as well as a psychological study of schizophrenic thinking. An attempt is under way to classify the different depressions and to determine their ideologies. Statistical studies are being made of psychoanalytic treatment results, and efforts are in progress to translate the principles and findings of psychoanalysis into preventive work. In keeping with another aspect of personality study is an effort to revise the Freudian scheme of personality structure.

Psychological researches include the clinical evaluation of modern psychological testing procedures, a project to establish the clinical value of the Lewinian topological psychology, an investigation of the mechanism of repression by experimental hypnosis and various psychological tests and methods, an inquiry into the differentiation of adjusted and maladjusted persons based on clinical histories and psychological testing results, and a study of the literature on the influence of emotions on memory.

Interest in children finds expression in specific researches having to do with children's psychological reactions to death, the reaction of superior children to children who are abnormal, the therapeutic use of marionettes, and a comparison of the personality structure and play techniques of adjusted and maladjusted children.

TOWSON, MD.

The Sheppard and Enoch Pratt Hospital

The Sheppard and Enoch Pratt Hospital is a voluntary mental hospital of some 300 beds, with a staff of 15 psychiatrists. It has long been recognized as one of the leading hospitals of the country and out of its wards and laboratories have come important research reports. Present studies are chiefly clinical in nature. While the laboratory facilities lend themselves readily to laboratory research, they are not particularly active in this respect.

The principal outside connection of this hospital is with the University of Maryland Medical School where three of its staff members are engaged in psychiatric teaching and assist in psychosomatic studies and give about one-third of the ordinary consultations to other departments.

The hospital gives psychiatric assistance to the Baltimore County Children's Agency and the State Traveling Clinics and, until recently, has similarly assisted the Baltimore public schools. Its library facilities, which include most of the psychiatric periodicals and standard texts, is supplemented by the libraries of the Henry Phipps Psychiatric Clinic and the Medico-Chirurgical Library of Baltimore. An effort is made to maintain complete volumes of important periodicals at one or another of these libraries and these publications are available to all of them.

The researches here tend toward studies of reaction pictures, particularly in ruminative tension states; etiological involvement of the auditory apparatus in various mental states; prognostic studies through the follow-up of discharged schizophrenic patients; and therapeutic studies directed toward the use of curare—protected convulsive shock and sleep therapy induced by barbiturates. In regard to the latter, there has been special interest in respiratory and circulatory alternations. With the acquisition of apparatus and necessary personnel, there is a growing interest in studies of the electrical reactions of the heart and brain and physical chemical constitution of the blood plasma.

VINELAND, N. J.

The Training School at Vineland, New Jersey

The Training School at Vineland, N. J., has long been recognized as a leading center of research in the field of mental deficiency and has many scientific contributions to its credit. It is a semi-private institution (school and custody) having some 430 children and adults plus an agricultural colony of about 100 boys and men. As an outgrowth of its interest in the spastic mental defective it has a department of 20 beds devoted to the training of spastic children of average normal intelligence and above. The school receives about two-thirds of its population as mentally defective state wards for training and has long had a close working relation with the various state institutions for the defective, the delinquent and others. It conducts clinics for spastic children in the state and has a close relation to local public schools which assist in providing necessary opportunities for the study of normal children. The records of all cases in the institution are filed in carefully indexed form in the research laboratory, where they can be easily selected for special study.

The research emanates largely from the research laboratory, which is chiefly a clinical psychological laboratory whose contributions come from studies of individual children. For several years it has been preoccupied with the measurement of social competence through the investigative use of a social maturity measuring scale developed there. It is also concerned with the experimental application of psychological testing devices to Selective Service registrants. There is an interest in gerontology, to the study of which the older cases in the institution lend themselves by very useful contrast with normal subjects of advanced years. Special studies are made from time to time as special case opportunities appear, as for example the study of motor disorders in relation to the etiology of mental deficiency. Besides its director, the laboratory has two assistants and from one to three fellows in training. Academic and laboratory courses in extension are offered at Rutgers University and at the Glassboro State Teachers College. Affiliation for academic credit is maintained with leading colleges and universities.

The Training School has close relationships with Duke University Hospital, with the Commission for Crippled Children in the New Jersey State Department of Health, with the A. Harry Moore School (public) for crippled children in Jersey City, N. J., and with a hospital for crippled children in Elizabethtown, Pa. It provides training for physical therapy in this field. It has a large medical consultant staff, chiefly from Philadelphia. The department for spastic cases has a part-time medical director and, through him, a close association with the Children's Rehabilitation Institute near Baltimore. It has also a psychologist in charge, and a physio-therapist. This department aims toward three objectives: the education of spastic children, their treatment, and research. It is interested in determination of the incidence of spastic paralysis in children. The clinical cases available for study include former patients who are the subject of continuous follow-up. Through the state clinics about 250 cases are seen each year. Extensive records, including films, are kept of all in-patients.

The Vineland Laboratory's library facilities are modest in extent, but carefully chosen, so that the collection includes most of the important psychological and psychiatric periodicals and the standard works. The library of the College of Physicians and Surgeons in Philadelphia is called on for additional service. Recourse is also had to other standard library sources, such as those of the University of Pennsylvania, the United States Public Health Service, the Army Medical Library, and others.

WASHINGTON, D. C.

Catholic University of America

Psychiatric research activities at the Catholic University were carried on for some years in the department of psychology under the direction of a psychiatrist who, in addition to his teaching and investigative work at the university, directed a psychiatric clinic for children and adults at the Providence Hospital in Washington. This clinic was recently transferred to the university campus to facilitate collaboration with the university's school of social service and as part of an enlarged program, established with financial aid from the Rockefeller Foundation, under which the department of psychology became the department of psychology and psychiatry. The new department functions as a graduate teaching and research center for the training of psychiatrists and non-medical workers in mental hospitals, clinics and other Catholic diocesan institutions and agencies. There is no medical school, but affiliations were established with Mount Hope Retreat, in Baltimore, and Providence Retreat, in Buffalo, private mental hospitals where physicians may secure psychiatric training and experience under the direction of the university's research professors of psychiatry. Training facilities are also afforded at St. Elizabeths Hospital, in Washington, as well as in the university psychiatric clinic.

The problems of research are often clinical in nature and are of varied scope. Considerable attention is given to studies in endocrine therapy. Current projects include Rorschach studies before and after hormone therapy, hyperactivity in children, play therapy, attitudinal studies in relation to learning, and various experimental techniques for the testing and measurement of intellectual and emotional development. For these studies there are available at the university adjunct clinical laboratories, including facilities for basal metabolic determinations. Biochemical facilities are afforded by coöperation of the biochemical laboratory in the department of chemistry. Frequent and original publications have emanated from the researches at this center. There is a substantial collection of psychiatric books and magazines in the university library, and access is had to other well stocked psychiatric and medical libraries in the city, such as the Library of the Surgeon General at the Army Medical Museum.

United States Public Health Service

An earlier report * dealt with research in St. Elizabeths Hospital, a large Federal hospital for mental disease (then an agency of the Department of the Interior, now under the Federal Security Administration), coördinated with the United States Public Health Service. The Mental Hygiene Division of the Public Health Service has directly under its jurisdiction the hospitals at Lexington, Kentucky, and Fort Worth, Texas, for the treatment of drug addiction and related problems; the psychiatric facilities at the 29 Federal institutions under the Bureau of Prisons (Department of Justice), of which the Medical Center for Federal Prisoners at Springfield, Missouri, is most outstanding; a mental hospital survey service; and a mental hygiene consultant service to state health departments to which Federal grants-in-aid are made for public health projects.

The hospital at Lexington gives special attention to the nature of drug addiction, its biophysical aspects, and its relation to the chemical structure of narcotic drugs. Some of these pharmacological studies are metabolic and deal with the economy of body water, serum cholinesterase, gaseous exchange, and the excretion of morphine and its derivatives.

Other studies are physiological and consider autonomic

---

* *Research in Mental Hospitals:* A Survey and Tentative Appraisal of Research Activities, Facilities and Possibilities in State Hospitals and Other Tax-Supported Institutions for the Mentally Ill and Defective in the United States. New York. 1938. The National Committee for Mental Hygiene. 151 p.

and hypothalamic functioning in addiction and on withdrawal, and the influence of narcotic drugs on cortical and hypothalamic electrical potentials. An attempt is being made to discover non-habit-forming substitute drugs, the influence of certain chemical structures (drugs) upon addiction, analgesic effectiveness of various drugs, and the influence of such drugs on the abstinence syndrome.

Psychological studies deal with the effect of situation upon autonomic response and methods for studying personality, especially by Rorschach tests, the differentiation of addicts, and tests of efficiency and emotions. Statistical studies are centered on the follow-up of treated cases. The library at the Lexington hospital includes the more important psychiatric periodicals, current and in bound form.

The hospital at Fort Worth is also focused on the addict. Rorschach studies are given special attention. Statistical studies of voluntary cases and of physician addicts are made here. A modification of the Craig test of syphilis is under way. Psychological studies deal with the factor of heredity in addiction, and special abilities and disabilities in addicts. Research on schizophrenia and other abnormal mental reactions in tuberculosis are also in progress. The library of this hospital includes the better psychiatric periodicals, bound and current.

Four of the prison hospitals under the United States Public Health Service are giving attention to studies in psychopathology, group psychotherapy and group psychometrics. In addition, statistical, biochemical, and psychological studies are matters of research interest. While the library of the hospital at Springfield, Missouri, includes the better psychiatric literature, the headquarters library at Washington, with its special mental hygiene section and its translations of foreign articles, is available to the hospitals in the field, and there is an exchange arrangement with the libraries of the Surgeons General of the Army and Navy and the Congressional Library that renders their resources available also.

WAUWATOSA, WIS.

Milwaukee Sanitarium

The Milwaukee Sanitarium is a private hospital located in Wauwatosa. It accommodates about 147 patients representing a class that is better equipped culturally, economically and intellectually than the average. Research in this center is the product of the individual interests of the staff members, but the staff is so selected that this interest is constant. While the motives of the sanitarium's activities are primarily therapeutic, research and study are encouraged, and the management has devoted some funds for this purpose.

Seven scientific papers have emanated from this center during the past three years, and there is an increasing interest in research problems. There are ties with two medical schools. The medical director is a trustee of Marquette University, and the chief psychiatric consultant of the sanitarium is lecturer in psychiatry at the University of Illinois. The Milwaukee County Hospital for Mental Diseases is nearby.

The laboratories of the sanitarium are designed primarily for the clinical needs of patients, the resources of nearby general hospitals being called on as needed. The research possibilities are thus oriented along clinical lines. The library facilities are centered on specific psychiatric periodicals, although other library facilities in Milwaukee offer practically everything else in the way of psychiatric references.

CHAPTER VIII
General Considerations and Conclusions

QUITE aside from the reflections as to the quality or breadth of the individual research centers, to which a survey of this sort may give rise, one may ask of oneself as one reviews these case stories: "What do they tell me about American psychiatry, American medicine, American science or the philosophy of the American people?" This question becomes even more insistent to those who have dwelt with this material during its preparation or who have had an opportunity of talking at first-hand with those who are directing the destinies of American psychiatry. There are many different philosophies, perspectives, ambitions, and concepts of what is important, and these may appear by implication in individual studies, or by a comparison of one center with another, but often they do not stand out in the printed line. There would seem to be some value, therefore, in setting forth some of these between-the-lines phases of psychiatric research.

Probably the most striking conclusion in this respect comes from seeing the material as a whole. This material shows that while in no one place is it fully expressed in the aggregate, American psychiatry has revealed a very great—almost complete—breadth of scope and interest. It is seriously concerned about the whole range of human living, because from the moment of conception and on into the far reaches of his succeeding generations man gets into trouble and, as a result, disturbs himself and his surroundings. These behavior troubles of man as a person are no longer believed to be mystically imposed or the result of some imaginary "construct" beyond his control, whereby man's participation in and his opportunity for improvement can be evaded. Man is accepting the fact that his troubles are caused by natural factors, often to be sure unknown, that he may hopefully investigate and

137

modify to his advantage. And so he is looking to psychiatry, which has come to see these factors magnified in order to achieve a better understanding of even his lesser troubles. Man looks to medicine, with its tradition of melioration, to show him ways out of his dilemmas, and so psychiatry, with a magnifying glass in one hand and antidotes in the other, is sleuthing man out as he bends his steps, often seemingly at great pains, toward getting into trouble.

One cannot study the works of the Vocational Adjustment Bureau, Institute of General Semantics, Riggs Foundation and the anthropological studies conducted under the Scottish Rite research program, without developing a consciousness of the critical effort to follow human function wherever it may lead scientific investigation. Even without considering the researches themselves, a great variety of institutions show the same tendency toward polymorphism—the Children's Rehabilitation Center, the Psychoanalytic Institute, Judge Baker Guidance Center and others. Even lesser functional differences, such as the acceptance of committed patients on the one hand and voluntary patients on the other, provide special opportunities and limitations to the research projects that are undertaken, and yet throughout the breadth of scope characterizing these projects there is not an even distribution of interest commensurate with the importance of the problems.

Psychiatry, itself a frontier, has its own frontiers and hinterlands. There are great concentrations and duplications of effort in certain spheres, whereas in others the attention given is meager. Where psychiatry has functioned for a long time one finds a greater concentration of attention; where it is branching out into new fields many of the studies undertaken are really unique. It is also very evident that the focus of attention of one decade may be virtually supplanted by another focus in a succeeding decade. Shock therapy is one of the most manifest current preoccupations, while studies of the effects of hidden infection, so imposing twenty years ago, have almost no place at the present time. Psychosomatic medicine, on the other hand, promises soon to become a major force. Other organic determinants—vitamin deficiency, fatigue, sleep, endocrine disorders, other nutritional disturbances, habits and tics and the normal reactions to emotion, fear and anger—seem to be given minor places in spite of their established relation to behavior deviations.

There is a disturbing paucity of research in the field of mental deficiency, considering the extent of its incidence and its social effects. This parallels the related paucity of competent personnel in that field. Cultural and anthropological conditions, while long recognized as potent determinants of human behavior, are only now beginning to be taken seriously in psychiatry, though still not very extensively.

Many criticisms have been directed against psychiatry for its rigidity, its tardiness of progress, its lack of scientific critique and of scientific development. In so far as these criticisms are justified, they are the expression of the institutionalizing forces of isolation of its major clinical resource, the large mental hospital, and also of the immensity of the job to be done and the limited resources with which to do it. Attempts to explain differences between various professional groups as an expression of a different quality of human beings has never had much validity. On the other hand, the mental hospital has not had the close association with medical schools, nor the well developed representation in the medical faculty, that has characterized some other branches of medicine. Present conditions indicate a change in that respect. Withal, these odds against psychiatry have allowed it, as shown by its research preoccupations, to consider some of the realities in its job that other branches of medicine could more easily ignore. Nowhere else is medicine so concerned with social service, the refinement of historical data, and integration with community functions generally. Nowhere else can the everyday living of the convalescent be ignored with greater difficulty. At the same time the different psychiatric centers vary greatly in their community ties. In some places the hospital is very much of a community institution, whereas in others it means little locally and derives no more of its patients from nearby areas than from a distance. This local tie has, however, been found highly valuable to research. It has provided local funds, local normal controls and local participation in experiments in controlling the social influences bearing on the disorder or on rehabilitation.

A study of the research activities of psychiatry shows that psychiatry is by no means resistant to progress or gullible in its acceptance of innovations. It was but a short time after initial reports were issued about each of the shock therapies that these therapies were being applied clinically and investigated both for their therapeutic value and for their by-effects. In many fields a sizeable accumulation of scientific data has been made through the efforts of the graduate student inspired and encouraged by the interest of the seasoned faculty member. In psychiatry this holds true to a degree also, but often the hospital that serves as a training center for graduate students is quite a distance from the city where the academic work is done, or the student may have no academic connection. Psychologists and psychiatric social workers, in addition to psychiatrists, have pursued special studies of psychiatric problems in this way, and on occasion there have been other participants, such as theological students. The university's attention to scientific questions and procedure and the hospital's preoccupation with practical services combine to produce research investigations that come closer to helping man with his troubles than would be the case without this twofold influence.

Psychiatric research is determined so much by individual interest that the trend in one center reappears in another center when a staff member changes his connections. There are centers in which, regardless of changes in staff, a certain trend will continue, but this is not generally the case. The center that became a veritable hive of activity under one leader finds itself inactive under another, or the activity may change its direction. In one instance valuable biochemical facilities reflecting an earlier period of research interest rest under lock and key awaiting future use, while other types of investigation flourish. Some investigators make a fetish of research and then look upon it as a badge of respectability, to be encouraged or stimulated for that reason. They may look askance at discoveries coming from the wards, the administrative offices or the classroom as being less respectable, regardless of their value to humanity. Any clinical techniques, administrative procedures or teaching methods, respectively, are put in a lower caste.

On the other hand, some find such considerations of little or no importance compared with the thrill of a slight success in the pursuit of an intriguing question, whatever its place. An iota of truth is its own sufficient reward. Some look with suspicion upon the inquisitive visitor who may reveal secrets upon which may depend the glory of priority of discovery. It is remarkable that in the psychiatric field such attitudes have been rare and never gross. Some investigators just seem to grope about for research projects, apparently lacking a great configuration of their field by which gaps become apparent. Others find tantalizing unknowns in everything they touch. Every psychiatric case, no matter how successfully handled, has its unknowns, so that not a great amount of inquisitiveness is necessary to discover grist for the research mill. It is evident in some instances that the imagination and philosophy underlying a piece of research emanate from an associate who has little time or inclination for research himself, but passes on his ideas as a stimulus to others. One man prides himself on doing this as his peculiar function.

It is not always this inquisitiveness that is behind the research drive, but at times rather an urge to prove something that intuition has dictated, and this urge to prove appears even in the titles of some research projects and publications. Fortunately, such an attitude is not always unproductive and is balanced by a reciprocal endeavor in some one else to prove the opposite. Many prejudices of this sort accompany the investigation of shock therapy. There is no question that in the eyes of the profession, and the public also, research productivity is something of a label and evidence of superiority, and not infrequently specious claims of research activity are made in order to achieve status. This contrasts markedly with the attitude of some other centers that are really giving more attention to research, but that have such a high critique of research that they hesitated to offer themselves for inclusion in this study. It is, therefore, not to be expected that the least of these included in this study is just above the best of those omitted. It is rather somewhat below.

Visits to many research centers elicited two extreme types of research preoccupation. Some literally love their instruments, others their theories. There are those who must have the latest embellishments and who can then produce abundantly in comfort. Others with the crudest equipment and quarters do outstanding work.

There is a great difference also in the eagerness to publish. Some preliminary reports are in reprint form before the study has completed its first stage. Others have accomplished important research results that have not been published because some details need further refinement.

Attempts have been made to recapture certain intangibles by showing the informal relationships that exist between various research centers or between such centers and other helpful facilities. Such a presentation must at best be incomplete, for important contacts are often isolated instances rather than continuing cooperation, and often over long distances. Taken as a whole, all these research centers are mutually supporting and the eye of one center tends to be focussed on the developing step in another center in order to be ready for the succeeding step in the progressive unfolding of the story of the mentally ill. Some places with many patients complement those with rich technical resources.

In considering the financial backing of research projects it must be kept in mind that the aggregate of monies spent for research is a very inadequate measure of the value of the time, effort and materials devoted to research. A very high proportion of the professional time spent in searching for new facts is a contribution of the research workers themselves, taken out of their off-duty hours or set aside from the hours of private psychiatric and neurological practice.

Some research centers are to all intents and purposes laboratories of ethical pharmaceutical and other commercial companies and are financed by them as they might be in the companies' own plants, but they are more effective when decentralized, because of the availability of clinical cases.

With the extensive periodical publications available in the psychiatric field as well as in other branches of medicine (there are some 12 regular psychiatric periodicals) and the continuous output of bound books, some research centers have given up the effort to maintain their own library resources to any degree of completeness, knowing that they can never be complete, and they have tended rather to look toward the pooling of library material with other branches of medicine and with other institutions geographically nearby.

There is a general tendency among those responsible for the organization and administration of institutions to think in absolute standards. A state mental hospital, they hold, should be set up so and so, under this or that state authority —state departments of welfare, health or mental hygiene, and all other forms are implied to be wrong. Or, psychiatry in a medical school should be set up as a separate department or should be set up in combination with neurology, or should be subordinate to internal medicine. Or again, psychiatric patients should be segregated or they should be dealt with as a part of the general patient population of a general hospital. Often the disadvantages of standardization are not apparent, but a study of the research activities under one pattern as contrasted with another shows that our knowledge has been enriched by these variations.

One of the outstanding developments in the field of psychiatric research at present on the up-grade is the interest in psychosomatic medicine and the movement of much psychiatric research from the locus of the psychotic to that of the neurological or general medical patient. Since this tendency is related to the appeal for the return of the family physician, it is expected that it will continue and that it will bring about a closer relationship between psychiatry and the other branches of medicine than has heretofore existed.

All in all it is evident that the expenditure of psychiatric time and brainpower and of money, often from the investigator's own pocket, is very considerable. About most of this expenditure one can have no qualms—even allowing for disagreement. Much of such effort, however,—chiefly the effort of persons inexperienced in research—could be turned to better advantage for psychiatry and the investigator himself, were mature and widely experienced advice available to him from a scientific advisory board composed of persons of unquestioned integrity and fully receptive to the new, who could assist the neophyte in appreciating the problems involved in pursuing his "hunches" and the methods available to hasten and point up his pursuit and to define the kinds of evidence that will be demanded to lead his studies to scientific conclusions. Such a group of sages would not only insure a greater economy of investigative effort but would tend to develop a more critical body of researchers in American psychiatry and perhaps identify the few who want to be expressive but not scientifically critical. Such an advisory function might well be a service to neophytes of the major scientific organization in American psychiatry, the American Psychiatric Association. Such a body might function to indicate the underworked aspects of psychiatry wherein research could be stimulated.

APPENDIX "A"

Annotated List of Current Research Projects

CALIFORNIA

California Department of Institutions, Sacramento

Research in insulin coma and various convulsive types of therapy for schizophrenia and other psychoses. Studies of convulsive therapy by electro-shock and electro-narcosis on experimental animals and on humans. Psychiatric social work studies of extramural care of mental patients.

Mount Zion Hospital, San Francisco

Studies of psychodynamic factors in schizophrenia, with special emphasis on ego development. Personality changes following substitution therapy in pre-adolescent eunuchoidism. Hypertension in one of identical twins.

Study of factors that enter into the success or failure of foster home and institutional placement of children. Personality adjustments of children in a model orphanage. An experiment in group treatment of neurotic adolescent girls.

Stanford University, San Francisco

Therapeutic use of alpha tocopherol (synthetic vitamin E) in progressive muscular atrophy, muscular dystrophies, and multiple sclerosis. Study of various factors responsible for the production of post-lumbar puncture headaches. Effect of production of an artificial adhesive leptomeningitis on the underlying parenchyma. Comparative histopathological study of the infantile and juvenile types of cerebromacular degeneration. Study of vascular changes in the pial vessels after cerebral trauma. Injury of the brain. Digestion of the brain. Vitamin deficiency in chicks.

Studies in psychosomatic medicine: Correlation of psychological inventories and test procedures with essential hypertension; correlation of psychological inventories and test procedures with peptic ulcer. Studies in pain. Emotional influences in atopic dermatitis. Psychoses associated with deafness. Clinical research in electroencephalography. Studies in reading disability.

145

Methods of determining blood alcohol concentration. Partition of alcohol between blood plasma and corpuscles. Relation between alcohol concentration of blood and urine after ingestion of alcohol. Alcohol and driving (a correlation of blood and alcohol concentration with various driving tests). Effect of various metabolites on alcohol metabolism.

University. of California, San Francisco

Medical Center
(In process of organization.)

Institute of Child Welfare, Berkeley
Growth Study of Adolescents: Behavior and motivation; development in adolescence; procedures and results in observational studies of social behavior; physiological changes in adolescence; development of interests and attitudes during adolescence; autonomic reactivity (as recorded by various instrumental methods) as related to personality characteristics.

The Berkeley Growth Study: Relationship of early mental scores to later mental development; individual case studies of children showing atypical patterns of mental growth; interrelationships among indices of maturity; item analysis of motor and mental tests with reference to socio-economic relationships and predictive significance.

The Guidance' Study: Studies in child guidance—a 20-year cumulative study (now in its 14th year) from birth, on physical, mental and personality development; evaluation studies on projective techniques (Rorschach, thematic apperception, play, among others); the meaning of differences in reputation among elementary school children; thumbsucking; parents' attitudes.

CONNECTICUT

Yale University, New Haven

Medical School
Methods of evaluating capacity for recovery in manic-depressive and schizophrenic patients: investigation of heredity, pre-psychotic personality, body build, serum lipoid pattern and mental status.

Investigations of obesity and malnutrition, particularly in the factors which control appetite: obesity in children; production of obesity in animals by hypothalamic lesions.

Blood lipoids in epilepsy. Relation between serum lipoid pattern and electroencephalographic findings. Evaluation of thyroid activity in agitated patients. Methods of measurement of blood and tissue iodine. Separation of organic iodine from inorganic iodine in blood. Iodine and thyroid disease. Distribution of iodine fractions in serum cells and spinal fluid. Investigations of organs that control blood lipoids: hypothalamus, liver, kidney, testicles and ovaries, pancreas. Serum protein and lipoid relations: nutrition, lymphogranuloma. Effects of temperature on thyroid activity.

Personality structure, personality development and personality adjustment. Psychopathic personalities. Experience and experiencing. Systematization: anancasm and paranoia.

Cumulative personality studies of clinical types. Masculinity-femininity studies. Intelligence and achievement. Level of aspiration. Visual problems, especially night vision. Eye potential studies. Emotional adjustment under conditions of tension.

Attitudes of unmarried expectant mothers. Post-partum personality disturbances. Electroencephalography and behavior.

Clinic of Child Development

Neuro-physiological studies of infant behavior, with special reference to autonomic functions in early months.

Clinical studies of behavior deviations and defects associated with cerebral injury and maldevelopment in infancy. Clinical aspects of child adoption.

Individual differences in developmental patterns of pre-school children. Symptomatic and dynamic aspects of ocular behavior in young children. Behavior deterioration and variance revealed by clinical examinations of young children.

Systematic studies of developmental morphology of infant behavior. Behavior characteristics of fetal-infant and full-term neonate. Dynamic and developmental aspects of behavior individuality as displayed in infants and pre-school children.

DISTRICT OF COLUMBIA

Catholic University of America, Washington

Physiological factors in the treatment of mental disorders. Special techniques of psychological therapy in mental disorders. Formal causality and the analysis of the general factor—a contribution to the mathematical analysis of mental symptoms, mental functions, and their interrelation.

Study of the intercorrelations of personality traits among a group of novices in religious communities. Study of the verbal and spatial elements in the synthetic sense. Construction of a test for measuring character traits. Effects of certain pharmacological preparations on the emotional life of normal individuals and those suffering from various mental disorders. Analysis of the mental and personality traits found in 250 major and minor seminarians.

A nomograph for obtaining tetrachoric correlation with determination of the numerical limits of the constants ordinarily involved in all equations for these correlations. Analysis of the intercorrelations of certain performance tests and an attempt to isolate the important factors involved and weight them so as to obtain the best possible measure of the functions underlying the tests.

Study of variability of performance on verbal and non-verbal tests, the significance of basal and maximal age in relation to grade status, the factorial composition of various performance tests, and of the Wechsler Bellevue Scale.

Factors that lead to the end of treatment in a child guidance case before the clinic thought treatment had been completed. Factors that led to fear of school in children and prompted their refusal to attend. A study of Catholic families that sought help from the child guidance clinic. An investigation of different types of children's humor. Play therapy and play analysis. An analysis of persistence. An analysis of reading interests and their relations to character traits.

United States Public Health Service, Washington

Public Health Service Hospital, Lexington, Ky.
The fate of morphine. Studies of morphine analgesia. Studies of the rôle of the hypothalamus and autonomic nervous system in morphine action and addiction. Studies of the addiction liability of a new synthetic analgesic.

Studies of the influence of morphine and morphine addiction on enzyme systems, on hormones, on water economy of the body, on personality (by means of the Rorschach test), on physiological responses to psychological stimuli.

Public Health Service Hospital, Fort Worth, Tex.
Addiction among physicians. Rorschach studies in drug addiction. Studies of voluntarily committed addicts. Special abilities and

disabilities in addicts. Heredity in addiction. " Craig's Test Modification." Schizophrenia and other abnormal mental reactions in tuberculosis.

GEORGIA

University of Georgia School of Medicine and University Hospital, Augusta
Blood pressure studies in convulsive therapy. Efforts to interpret the so-called psychopathic personality. Study of a new pyramidal tract sign. Studies in electric shock therapy.

ILLINOIS

Institute of General Semantics, Chicago
(Information not available.)

Institute for Psychoanalysis, Chicago
Studies of emotional factors in: Endocrine and metabolic disturbances (bulemia, frigidity, pituitary disorders, diabetes); skin disorders (urticaria, eczema, neuro-dermititis); cardio-vascular disorders (hypertension and hypotension); glaucoma.

Electroencephalograms and personality. Brief psychotherapy: application of psychoanalytic principles to general psychiatric problems. Microscopic study of dreams.

Loyola University and Cook County Hospital, Chicago
Study of carbohydrate metabolism in functional mental disorders. Studies of the functional psychoses in an attempt to isolate an anti-insulinic hormone. Experimental and clinical investigation of the effect of methyl guanidine sulphate.

Michael Reese Hospital, Chicago
Psychoanalytic studies of ambulatory schizophrenia. Studies of hypothalamic function in chronic encephalitis. Further studies in stimulation of the hypothalamus in the schizophrenic.

Physiological disturbances of cerebral vessels following head injury. Effect of so-called cortical and subcortical hypnotics on the human EEG as measured with cortical " H " leads. Psychosomatic studies of thyroid disturbances. Correlation of the dynamics of personality types and gastric secretion. Electrical anaesthesia in the human. Psychotherapy of migraine.

Rorschach response pattern in hysteria as differentiated from other neuroses and patients with somatic disorders. Rorschach and psychometric findings in children with allergy. Rorschach findings in children with petit mal convulsions, before and after hyperventilation. Personality findings as correlated with rate and quantity of gastric secretions. Rorschach findings in non-clinic groups of children, beginning in the nursery years.

Test studies: Stanford-Binet Scatter in relation to clinical evidence of personal instability; Goodenough drawing scale on children with certain clinical pictures; Vineland Social Maturity Scale, as a clinical aid in children referred for adoption.

Emotional aspects of reading disabilities in children. Psychology of the immigrant. Study of the problem of intellectual defenses.

Northwestern University, Chicago

Introversion-extroversion tests. Properties of the quasi visible spectrum. Properties of electrical waves used to produce convulsions in schizophrenics. Value of electric shock therapy. Changes in brain waves after electric shock therapy.

Studies in treatment of epilepsy by bromides: Relation of bromide in blood to that in urine; toxicity of dilantin; water metabolism in epilepsy; effect upon the brains of animals as the result of electrically produced convulsions.

Anticonvulsant drugs. A new method of measurement of bromide in the blood and saliva. Effects upon the nervous system of convulsions produced by metrazol and insulin. Effect of atmospheric compression upon the central nervous system—preliminary to a study of relation of blast to war neuroses.

Production of shock by acetyl cholin. Effect of bulbocapnin upon the central nervous system. Effect of lowering temperature upon respiration and heart action. Effect of convulsions on central nervous system. Lipase content of cerebrospinal fluid in catatonia and other cases of schizophrenia.

Threshold for binocular and monocular flicker fusion. Deterioration in epilepsy with an evaluation of deterioration scales. Effects of frontal lobe lesions on perception and higher mental functions. Personality and mental concomitants of bone maturity. Perceptual thresholds to complex forms and figures. Vibratory sensitivity. Relationships between motivational factors of "level of aspiration" and "degree of effort." Effect of cafeine and benzedrine on fatigue.

Studies in delinquencies, anthropologic, physiologic, psychologic and sociologic aspects.

University of Chicago, Chicago

Department of Medicine

Study of psychogenic factors in cases of emesis. Study of emotional factors in eczema, asthma, feeding problems. Studies of psychosomatic relations in endocrine disorders, in sexual disorders, and in headaches.

Clinical application of a test of imagination to neurotic children. Maternal rejection. Evaluation of experimental psychological investigation of the concepts of clinical psychiatry. Evaluation of handwriting analysis in the study of personality, with special reference to problems of diagnosis and prediction.

Electroencephalographic study of tumors and other intracranial conditions. Study of electrical phenomena in the brain following convulsions produced by shock.

Insulin inhibition in schizophrenic patients. Lipoid metabolism in various neuroses and psychoses. Physiological aspects of migraine.

Study of psychological aspects of schizophrenia; psychotherapy in schizophrenia; phantasy investigations in schizophrenia and schizophrenic thinking disorders.

Study of hallucinations in alcoholic psychoses and schizophrenia. Studies of behavioral effects of brain injuries in carefully selected neurosurgical patients by the use of new and by standard objective methods.

Evaluation of vocational tests and counselling processes. Follow-up study of physically handicapped patients following vocational testing and counselling.

Study of Kuhlman and Stanford-Binet tests on normal adults, students, organic cases. Variations in psychometric findings in children treated for emotional disturbances. Psychometric tests in epileptic patients.

Department of Anatomy

Investigation on the anatomy of the retina. Study of effect of stimulation and absence of stimulation on the degenerating neurons. Anatomical study of central nervous system of a case of complete transection of the spinal chord twenty-eight years before death.

Department of Pharmacology

Study of hibernation in relation to catatonia. Study of pharmacological control of lipoid metabolism, using the injection of acetyl

B-methyl choline as a method for producing changes in the lipoid content of the blood.

Department of Pathology
Investigation of nature of brain lipoids by immunological methods and principle of serological test for syphilis. Study of conditional reflexes and experimental neurosis in animals (production of asthma in the dog and influence of heredity and of vitamin deficiency on experimental production of neuroses).

Department of Psychology
Study of psychological changes in monkeys and apes with various segments of brain removed by operation. Study of mechanisms of hallucinations, especially those produced by the drug mescaline. Mechanisms involved in eidetic imagery and other sensory deceptions.

Orthogenic School
Nature of emotional rigidity in juvenile schizophrenia. Nature of the childhood personalities and social background of adult psychotics. Reactions of neurotic and normal children to frustration. Psychological factors involved in the blocking responses to emotionally provoking stimuli. Factors of emotionality and personality in reading deficiencies.

KANSAS

Menninger Sanitarium and Clinic and Southard School, Topeka
Rorschach studies in metrazol and somium amytal. Influence of emotions on memory. Analysis of sequence in the Rorschach test. Frustration experiments and Freudian mechanisms. Concept formation tests. Double personalities.

Emotional factors in hypertension. Short term psychotherapy of psychosomatic problems, with the data of the interview correlated with physiological changes. Short term anamnestic studies of cases of peptic ulcer. Psychoanalytic study of case of hypertension and peptic ulcer. Study of anorexia nervosa.

Modified psychoanalytic technique in the treatment of schizophrenia. Evaluation of the results of psychoanalytic treatment. Effect of a previous psychosis upon psychoanalytic treatment and personality structure. Analysis of the structure of the so-called psychopathic personality. Comparison of various psychological concepts in general psychology with psychoanalytic findings.

Methodological consideration of the concept of repression. Investigation of the relation of memory and emotional adjustment by use of Zeigarnik technique.

Psychiatric studies of "normal" individuals. Descriptive study of alcohol addiction. Study of somatic suicide. Psychology of the deaf. Analysis of schizophrenic drawings. Experimental production of anti-social behavior by the use of hypnosis. Psychological factors in twinships.

Ten year study of use of occupational therapy techniques in treatment of psychiatric patients, to determine effectiveness of occupational therapy, suitability of different types of personalities for occupational therapy, functions of hobbies, methods of teaching, etc.

KENTUCKY

University of Louisville, Louisville

Experimentation in teaching methods with medical students, including coöperative teaching with department of anatomy for first year students, with department of pathology for second year students, with department of medicine for third year students, and with internists in practice for fourth year students.

Study of effectiveness of psychiatric training of medical interns and residents rotating through the psychiatric service over the last eight years.

Experimentation with a nursery school set-up in a mental hygiene clinic. Evaluation of factors leading to improvement of children's behavior and parent-child relationships.

Evaluation of teachers' behavior in the classroom in terms of mental hygiene concepts. Electroencephalographic studies on preschool problem children.

Treatment of profound hypochondriasis by insulin. Investigations of functions of the frontal lobe. Hypnosis studies on general paretics. Rôle of factors underlying bromide addiction.

MARYLAND

Chestnut Lodge Sanitarium, Rockville

Studies of the effects of psychoanalysis on patients, the effects of patients undergoing analysis on other patients, and the relationship between patients, staff and other personnel with special reference to discernible trends influencing both individuals and groups.

Children's Rehabilitation Institute, Baltimore
Infantilization of birth injured children.

Johns Hopkins University, Baltimore

Department of Psychiatry and Henry Phipps Psychiatric Clinic
Studies in psychobiological laboratory. Studies on alcohol; skin resistance; nutrition; cyclical changes; epilepsy and electroencephalography. Study of conditioned reflexes and experimental neuroses. Analysis of case records. Motion picture study of catatonia.

Researches in dementia praecox: Evaluation of schizophrenics responding favorably to insulin treatment, comparative study; schizophrenic thinking among Navaho Indians in New Mexico; schizophrenic thinking and physical measurements; psychobiological researches on taste and appetite in schizophrenics.

Children's Psychiatric Service (Harriet Lane Home)
Study of frequency, age and sex incidence of specific complaints about children's behavior. Study of autistic disturbances of affective contact in small children. Play investigation and play therapy. Development of sex awareness and sex attitudes in children. Study of slurred comprehension of words.

Cultural implications of children's behavior problems. Influence of previous outside employment or professional career of mothers on mother-child relationships. Early resistance of children and its management. Study of parental misconceptions concerning child health and behavior. Review of books on child psychiatry to be recommended to physicians and parents.

The social calendar of the R. family: a day-by-day study of a maladjusted family for a one-year period, its behavior, social attitude, demands upon and cost to the community. Study of the psychiatric problems of children in a rural area. Continuing follow-up of a group of 700 children examined in 1930–32.

School of Hygiene and Public Health
Analysis of survey material in Mental Hygiene Study of Eastern Health District as to demographic facts and factors related to mental health problems.

Analysis of American and European statistics on the psychoses with special reference to the ratio between manic-depressive and schizophrenic psychoses in relation to social-economic status.

Study of records of mental hygiene clinic operated in conjunction with Well Baby Clinics of Eastern Health District, including "normal" pre-school children as well as "complaint cases." Study of sex rhythms in white and colored families on basis of histories obtained in this clinic.

Sheppard and Enoch Pratt Hospital, Towson

Applications of tests, such as the Rorschach, Hartford-Shipley scale, etc., to problems of reaction types; studies of thresholds of sensory perception in relation to problems of reaction types.

Clinical studies of personality types presenting: Obsessive ruminative tension states; morbid fear and anxiety; manic-depressive reactions, and psychopathic personality reactions. Psychiatric studies of accepted inductees in Army service.

Clinical studies of effects of stilbestrol on depressive states with suspension of menses. Physico-chemical studies of blood plasma. Possible applications of electroencephalography to study of emotional reactions in psychiatric patients. Determination of barbiturate concentration in the body fluids.

Therapeutic effects of sodium-amytal-induced sleep and of curare-protected convulsive shock on patients not responding to other therapy. Studies of immediate and remote effects of curare-protected convulsive shock therapy in relation to respiratory and circulatory changes. Effects of curare and curare-protected shock on blood chemistry. Efficiency of curare and related drugs in protecting patients from traumatic injury in convulsive shock therapy.

MASSACHUSETTS

Austen Fox Riggs Foundation, Inc., Stockbridge

Study of psychiatric services in New England colleges.

Beth Israel Hospital, Boston

Various psychological aspects of food problems in relation to diet, obesity, etc.; convalescent problems, with special reference to anxiety; emotional factors in chronic illness; various problems presented in general hospitals as seen through consultation service; relationships of family agencies to a psychiatric clinic.

Boston City Hospital, Boston

Therapy of convulsive disorders; chemical basis of anti-convulsant activity of drugs; syphilis of the nervous system; disorders of muscular movements.

Migraine. Sociological, hereditary and biochemical studies of convulsive disorders.

Electroencephalography in electrical activity of the human cortex in various age groups, convulsive disorders, and other diseases of the nervous system. Differentiation of brain waves. Biochemistry in relation to the electrical activity of the cerebral cortex in humans. Alcoholism and suicide.

Children's Hospital, Boston

Continuing researches into psychological aspects of cerebral injuries and infections and the effects of acute or chronic disease upon mental development and behavior; study of after effects of lead poisoning from the psychological standpoint.

Habit Clinic for Child Guidance and Tufts College Medical School, Boston

Study of adoptions. Study of the direct and indirect effects of the war upon children. Study of "popularity" of children in the lower classes of the public school system.

Judge Baker Guidance Center, Boston

Analysis of 500 delinquent cases treated at the clinic, the treatment given, and the results after an interval of five years.

Studies of abnormal personalities; of the psychoanalytic aspects of rejected children; of runaway children; of the early psychodynamic aspects of schizophrenia.

Massachusetts Department of Mental Health, Boston

(Research project ended October 1, 1941.)

Massachusetts General Hospital, Boston

(Normal research activities suspended with onset of war. Superseded by research projects in military psychiatry.)

McLean Hospital, Waverley

(Information not available.)

Peter Bent Brigham Hospital, Boston

Investigation of emotional reactions of patients to ward-round teaching and to illness of all types.

Studies of intellectual and emotional behavior in patients suffering from various deliria; physiological studies of these patients in respect to certain functions of cerebral metabolism.

Supreme Council, 33°, Scottish Rite, Northern Masonic Jurisdiction, Boston

(See Chapter VII, pages 104–107.)

MICHIGAN

Henry Ford Hospital, Detroit

Main research interests integrated with general conduct and maintenance of division of neuropsychiatry considered as an experiment in a general hospital setting. Secondary research projects include: Special studies of psychoneuroses; a study of the shock therapies; and special studies pertaining to the intravertebral disk, including epidurography.

Wayne University and Eloise Hospital, Detroit

Studies in hypnosis. Experiments in metrazol, insulin and electric shock therapies. Prognostic studies of psychological performance and muscular-coördination characteristics of tuberculous patients.

MINNESOTA

University of Minnesota and Minnesota General Hospital, Minneapolis-St. Paul

Minnesota Multiphasic Personality Schedule. Emotional factors in gastric ulcer syndrome, using both Minnesota Multiphasic Personality Schedule and conventional psychiatric interviews. Use of curare in convulsive states. Treatment of Parkinsonism with hyoscine, rabellon, quinine and bellabulgara.

Metastatic tumors of the nervous system. Structure of small cerebral blood vessels in hypertension and in chronic degenerating conditions. Effects of anemia on central nervous system. Effects of sulfonimide drugs on central nervous system. Effect of vitamin B$_6$ on organic psychosis. Physiological recovery pattern of electrical skin resistance after experimentally produced stress.

MISSOURI

Neurological Hospital, Kansas City

Studies of psychotic manifestations in the older patient. Correlation of findings and observations in the toxic delirious reactions of old age.

Washington University, St. Louis

Application of the Strong Vocational Interest Test for selection of desirable candidates for medical training; application of this test to physicians in various medical specialties and to social case workers.

Conditioned reflexes in humans using vaso-motor responses as an indicator. Functions of the frontal lobes and of the corpus callosum of carnivors and monkeys. Psychological and psychiatric changes following therapeutic surgical lesions of the frontal lobes in humans. Functions of the brain stem and the interrelations between brain stem and the cortex in carnivors. Study of the mechanism of concussion.

Cytological studies on the pineal gland and on gliomas. Analysis of stimulation and responses of optic nerve. Potential differences between cortex, corpus striatum and colliculus. Sources of brain waves.

Electroencephalographic changes during artificial hyperpyrexia. Use of alpha-tocopherol and various factors of the B complex in diseases of the central nervous system. Etiology and pathology of encephalomyelitis. Treatment of paresis with pharmacological shock.

Personality changes following surgical operations. Study of a group of patients on medical wards who are showing disturbances, on the Shipley-Hartford Scale. Clinical study of folie a deux. Occupational incapacities in social agency clients. Psychological problems involved in foster home care. The cultural problem of psychoses among negroes. Psychodynamic factors of post-partum psychosis in negroes.

NEBRASKA

University of Nebraska Medical School, Omaha
Continuing studies with curare and curare-like drugs combined with metrazol and electro-shock therapy; electro-shock therapy in depressive states; use of magnesium sulphate in convulsive shock therapy.

Combined aldarsone and fever therapy in the treatment of paretic dementia.

Electroencephalographic studies in paretic dementia and in psychotic and traumatic cerebral conditions.

NEW JERSEY

Training School at Vineland
Manual of Vineland Social Maturity Scale, giving directions for use of scale, normal standardization, feebleminded validation, and summary of experimental studies.

Further application studies with Vineland Social Maturity Scale: Social competence of blind children; social competence of the mentally disordered; social competence of negroes; growth studies in social competence with normal subjects and with feebleminded subjects.

Growth studies on the intelligence of the feebleminded. Studies on etiology of mental deficiency. Studies on symptom complex clinical varieties of mental deficiency. Motor equilibrium in relation to etiological type of mental deficiency. Clinical case studies of special types of mental deficiency, special disability, and behavior disorders.

Coöperation on problems of psychology in relation to national defense.

NEW YORK

Albany Hospital and Albany Medical College, Albany

Investigation of proceeding concerning memory; concerning cerebral blood supply in the aged; concerning skin temperatures in depressive patients before and after treatment; concerning the preservation of adequate functional levels during anoxia.

Committee for the Study of Sex Variants, New York

(Information not available.)

Hillside Hospital, New York

Electrocardiographic studies in connection with electric shock therapy. Study of post-partum reactive mental disorders in relation to the menstrual cycle.

Jewish Board of Guardians, New York

Studies of primary behavior disorders; of runaways; of criteria for institutionalization. Study of case work use of fees. Follow-up study of child-guidance cases of selected years.

Lifwynn Foundation, New York

Comparative study of electroencephalographic patterns in attention and cotention.

Differentiation of oculo-motor patterns in affecto-symbolic dissociations (neurosis, individual and social) as contrasted with the organism's primary biological adaptation to the environment.

Investigation of metabolic alterations in the two patterns of adaptation.

Extension of instrumental research in respiratory patterns characterizing alterations in attentional adaptation.

Investigation of possible application of mechanical adjuncts in effecting the required shift to altered adaptive (attentional) pattern.

Continuing laboratory investigation of human relations in their daily living expressions.

Mount Sinai Hospital, New York

Department of Neurology—Psychiatric Division
Psychosomatic factors in the psychoses. Problems in epileptics. Neuroses in recent immigrants. Autonomic disturbances in psychoneurotics. The Lines-Test for the diagnosis of psychoneuroses. Classification of psychosomatic disorders.

Character types, predisposing and precipitating factors in peptic ulcer and in essential hypertension. Menopausal disturbances from a psychiatric point of view. Psychiatric disturbances in brain tumors. Early aphasic disturbances in brain tumors. Temperature studies in hypoglycemic states.

Respiratory types in the psychoneuroses (by a new method); study of respiratory variations in relation to sleep (by a new method); methods of induction of states of partial sleep in relation to analytic treatment.

Factors influencing occupational choice and adjustments. Finger painting; painting analysis; color therapy; personality structure in nurses.

Department of Pediatrics—Children's Health Class
Relation of graphology, palmistry and the Rorschach test. Study of precocious puberty. Studies of capillaries in problem children. Analyses of the constancy of the I.Q. and reasons for its deviation.

New York Hospital—Cornell University Medical Center, New York

Payne Whitney Psychiatric Clinic
Influence of emotional factors in various physical disorders; influence of emotions on gastric functions and other physiological functions.

Studies of leucocytosis in psychopathological disorders. Studies of the menstrual cycle and ovarian functions. Biochemical studies in various psychological disorders. Experimental studies on hypothermia. Neurophysiological investigations (electroencephalographic and electromyographic).

Psychopathological studies in the late-life period. Study of the family in relation to sickness and health care. Various investigations of anxiety and fear in young children. Catholicism and personality disorders.

Westchester Division, White Plains

Continuing studies of shock therapy and results obtained. Psychological studies of shock therapy, before and after treatment, to determine mental efficiency.

Follow-up study of psychoneurotic women patients admitted over a period of ten years, with inventory of results shown following discharge from hospital.

Electrocardiographic and electroencephalographic studies of psychiatric reactions in inebriates and other mental patients.

New York Infirmary for Women and Children, New York

Relation of type of adolescence to early childhood. Relation of school achievement to early childhood. Continuing dynamic study of two groups of children through adolescence. Studies of adoption. Anthropological studies.

Studies of activity pattern, its persistence and modifiability, its relation to personality, development, etc. Devising and improving tests appropriate for each age level as an aid in following the child's activity pattern and type of responses to (a) overcoming obstacles, (b) removal and restoration of object of gratification. Application of latter test in evaluation of child's ability to adjust and type of care needed.

New York Post Graduate Hospital and Medical School, New York

Analysis of behavior problems in children. Studies in intra-family relations, with special reference to psychopathological factors in divorce.

New York State Department of Mental Hygiene, Albany

Evaluation of results obtained by electric shock therapy. Parole and family care. Racial distribution of admissions to state schools. A comprehensive history of the care of the insane in the State of New York.

New York Vocational Adjustment Bureau for Girls, New York*
Value of MacQuarrie test as a diagnostic instrument. Value of the
level-efficiency analysis in the borderline and low average cases.
Level-efficiency analysis of the Terman scale and its relation to
scatter.

Standardization of tests used in like units to make them imme-
diately comparable. Study of the relationship between the Shipley-
Hartford scale and the different levels of intelligence.

Pinewood, Katonah
Electric convulsive treatments; statistical studies as to their efficacy
in the various psychoses. Treatment of alcoholism by means of
insulin and glucose. Effects of sub-comatose doses of insulin on
various psychotic conditions.

Stony Lodge, Ossining
Critical study of clinical records of 500 patients treated at Stony
Lodge between 1925 and 1941. The nature of the therapeutic
effects of electro-shock therapy. Problems in psychosomatic
medicine.

Syracuse Psychopathic Hospital and Syracuse University, Syracuse
Correlation of blood pressure and spinal fluid pressure after
intravenous amphetamine. Combined treatment with barbiturates
and amphetamine and modifications; use of amphetamine sulfate
as an analeptic index; treatment of alcoholic psychoses with
amphetamine; use of sodium delvinal as a barbiturate sedative; use
of endocrine products and other forms of therapy.

Treatment of encephalitis. Treatment of epilepsy. Psychosomatic
relations in a general and in a mental hospital. Comparison of
cases of suicide in a general hospital and in a mental hospital.
Treatment of involutional psychoses, including the use of endo-
metrial biopsies in evaluating the physiological response.

Mental hygiene of childhood. Occupational therapy and play techniques; re-educational function of the play group in the child
guidance clinic; study of the comparative reaction in two groups
of children with conduct disorders to drawing and music tech-

---

* In April 1942 this Bureau became the Vocational Adjustment Division of
the National Committee for Mental Hygiene for the purpose of national consultation and advice in this field. For local services in New York City, it
functions under the direction of its own Board, and is concentrating its
attention on the rehabilitation of mentally handicapped men for purposes of
increased manpower.

niques; additional factors in juvenile delinquency. Continuing studies of special mental disabilities in speech, reading and writing in relation to conduct disorders.

OHIO

University of Cincinnati and Cincinnati General Hospital, Cincinnati

Department of Anatomy
Investigations of the relations of the central nervous system to internal glands in metabolic and visceral disease.

Department of Physiology
Studies on Belladonna derivatives in Parkinsonism. Clinical trial of new dilantin derivatives in epilepsy. Study of Eugene, a dilantin-treated epileptic.

Department of Biochemistry
Studies of cholinergic substances; relation of vitamin B_1 to cholinergic substances.

Department of Pharmacology
Pharmaco-dynamics of drugs actively used at present in psychiatry.

Department of Psychology
Rorschach studies in connection with brain surgery cases and with intensive vitamin feeding to malnourished and retarded children. Study of the production, persistence, transmission, and removal of psychogenically induced convulsive states in the white rat. Analysis of the stages in recovery from the fatigue effects of continuous mental work. Compilation of material on modes of propaganda, selection of personnel, methods of building morale in German recruits, and of controlling Nazi spies in America.

Laboratory of Neuropathology
Cerebral blood flow in health and disease. Electroencephalographic studies of alcoholism and toxemias of pregnancy. Study of various aspects of vitamin B problem in relation to mental disorders.

Children's Hospital
Investigations on the natural history of human and experimental poliomyelitis. Investigations of the rôle of age in resistance to involvement of the nervous system by certain viruses; rôle of nutrition in resistance of nervous system to involvement by various viruses. Toxoplasmic encephalitis (incidence, specific diagnosis and chemotherapy).

Child Guidance Home
Diagnostic and prognostic significance of the differences between the intelligence quotient and the social quotient. Critical study of environmental influences responsible for behavior disorders of children based on analysis of 350 cases. Effect of growth hormone in influencing height of undersized children. Effect of large doses of gonadotrophic substance on epiphyseal closure. Personality evaluation studies.

May Institute for Medical Research
Relationship of pituitary gland to somnolence and sleep. Influence of various pharmacological materials on the hematoencephalic barrier. Influence of dyes on production of convulsions in the new-born. Influence of vitamins and metabolic changes on the convulsive threshold in various species. Influence of various types of vitamin deficiency on response to noise.

Longview State Hospital
Electroencephalographic studies of various types of mental disease and of post-encephalitic cases. Effects of drugs on peripheral blood flow in psychiatric patients. Levels of blood adrenalin and shock therapies. Effects of various synthetic and natural estrogens in involutional melancholias, with parallel studies of behavior and vaginal smears. Relation between brain waves and autonomic changes during the menstrual cycle. Effect of barometric pressure on resistance of patients to shock doses of insulin.

Western Reserve University, Cleveland

City Hospital
Clinico-pathological studies in cases of chronic flaccid hemiplegia. Electroencephalographic studies on old age, Alzheimer's and Pick's disease. Electroencephalographic studies on cases of hypoparathyroidism. Mental and physical capacities after right cerebral hemispherectomy. Post-traumatic encephalopathy. Better therapies for epilepsy.

Cleveland Guidance Center
(Information not available.)

OREGON

University of Oregon Medical School, Portland
Experimentation in providing child guidance clinic services for rural areas. Experimentation in aiding general medical practitioners in treating psychoneuroses. Clinical studies of suicide.

PENNSYLVANIA

Elwyn Training School, Elwyn
Studies in metabolism and immunological research.

Gladwyne Colony, Gladwyne
Studies in colloidal chemistry, physical chemistry, physiology and psychology.

Jefferson Medical College, Philadelphia
Problems of out-patient hypothalamic functions and emotions, anxiety neuroses, impotence, and convulsions. Biochemical and physical studies of nervous function.

Philadelphia Child Guidance Clinic, Philadelphia
Study of refinements in the nature of the therapeutic process, both with children and parents. Parents' participation in psychotherapy. Adolescent therapy. Psychology of the child under three.

Philadelphia General Hospital, Philadelphia
Study of pigment cells in the brain. Abnormalities of cerebral vessels and anoxemia.

Temple University School of Medicine, Philadelphia
Physico-chemical changes associated with convulsions. Factors influencing the convulsive reaction. Vestibulo-ocular reflex mechanisms. Cortical innervation of internal organs.

Electrocardiographic studies of psychotic patients. Rorschach studies of personality characteristics of failing students.

University of Pennsylvania—Pennsylvania Hospital, Philadelphia
Clinical and follow-up studies of electro-shock therapy; studies of insulin shock treatment. Electroencephalographic studies following electro-shock treatment; electroencephalographic studies of cortical changes and other conditions. Evaluation of migraine treatment. Studies of psychosomatic disorders. Psychiatric aspects of military medicine.

Effect of drugs and chemicals on synaptic connections and on nerve conduction. Microtechnic for determination of oxygen exchange in tissues, oxygen tension in intercellular fluids of brain.

Quantitative measurement of cerebral blood flow. Stimulation of neurons of respiratory center by means of various agents. Balances between reflexes and direct central effects in control of respiration. Influence of different anesthetic drugs on central nervous activities. Neurophysiology of spinal cord.

RHODE ISLAND

Butler Hospital, Providence

Study of memory changes in shock treatment. Determination of metabolic and respiratory changes under emotional stimuli in schizophrenic patients. Organic brain changes involving verbal and judgmental changes in frontal lobectomy. Rorschach characteristics of organic aphasias. Psychological and localization tests in Pick's disease.

Emma Pendleton Bradley Home, East Providence

Clinical studies in electroencephalography, with special reference to behavior problems in children. Clinical studies of schizophrenia in childhood.

Follow-up studies on children diagnosed as schizophrenic or schizoid who have been under observation for a period of years.

Studies of the effects of drugs on the behavior of children. Now investigating benzedrine sulphate, phenobarbital, and synthetic vitamin E (alpha-tocopherol).

Preparation of symptom index covering all problem children admitted to institution.

Indexing incidence of asphyxiating diseases in all problem children and correlation with types of behavior clinically observed and with electroencephalograms.

TENNESSEE

Vanderbilt University School of Medicine, Nashville

Epidemiological study of psychiatric and mental health problems in a rural area by means of experimental clinic associated with county health department.

Pharmacological research: studies of effects of anti-convulsant drugs.

VIRGINIA

Tucker Hospital, Richmond

Investigation of albinism. Neuropathological investigation of patients who have received shock treatment, and clinical evaluation of shock treatment. Clinical pathological study of torulosis histolytica. Investigation of the forms and value of fever therapy in neuropsychiatry.

Westbrook Sanatorium, Richmond

Clinical studies in shock therapy: use of codeine in treatment of morphinism and of sodium chloride in delirium tremens.

Diagnostic studies: correlation of blood, alcohol and behavior variations in hypoglycemia; symptomatic significance of achlorhydria; correlation of alcoholism and pellagra.

WISCONSIN

Milwaukee Sanitarium, Wauwatosa

Surgery in the lives of psychiatric patients. Masculine-feminine factors in the lives of psychiatric patients. Reactions of patients to deaths in their families. Etiological factors in dementia precox. Constitutional asthenia. Geography of some mental hygiene implications in the set-up of state governments. Follow-up on 111 ambulatory depressed patients after 14 years. A chart for use in recording reactions of patients in insulin shock therapy. Advances in shock therapy.

APPENDIX " B "

Roster of Professional Personnel Engaged in Research

CALIFORNIA

California Department of Institutions, Sacramento

Aaron J. Rosanoff, M.D., Director.

Nathan Sloate, Supervisor of Extramural Care.

Jacob P. Frostig, M.D., Department of Psychiatry, University of California Medical School.

Max Mason, Ph.D., Sc.D., Member of Executive Council, California Institute of Technology.

M. S. Plesset, Ph.D., Physicist, California Institute of Technology.

G. W. Potapenko, Physicist, California Institute of Technology.

A. van Harreveld, M.D., Physiologist, California Institute of Technology.

C. A. G. Wiersma, M.D., Physiologist, California Institute of Technology.

Mount Zion Hospital, San Francisco

Jacob Kasanin, M.D., Chief, Psychiatric Service.

Joseph C. Solomon, M.D., Associate Chief, Psychiatric Service.

Sophia Mirviss, M.D., Research Fellow in Psychiatry.

Meyer M. Friedman, M.D., Cardio-Vascular Research Laboratory.

Gerson R. Biskind, M.D., Department of Pathology.

Pearl L. Axelrod, Clinic Psychiatric Social Worker.

Benjamin Bonapart, Superintendent of Homewood Terrace.

Stanford University, San Francisco

George S. Johnson, M.D., Professor of Neuropsychiatry.

Henry W. Newman, M.D., Assistant Professor of Neuropsychiatry.

Leon J. Whitsell, M.D., Resident in Neuropsychiatry.

Frederick L. Reichert, M.D., Professor of Surgery.

Hale F. Shirley, M.D., Assistant Professor of Pediatrics and Psychiatry.

Mary Isabel Preston, M.D., Assistant Clinical Professor of Pediatrics.

Frederick A. Fender, M.D., Clinical Instructor in Surgery and Neuropsychiatry.

Ernest G. Lion, M.D., Clinical Instructor in Neuropsychiatry.

169

170   RESEARCH IN MENTAL HOSPITALS

John F. Card, M.D., Clinical Instructor in Neuropsychiatry.
William M. Cameron, M.D., Clinical Instructor in Neuropsychiatry.
Robert S. Turner, Ph.D., Instructor in Anatomy.

University of California, San Francisco

Medical Center

Karl M. Bowman, M.D., Medical Superintendent, Langley Porter Clinic; Professor of Psychiatry.
E. W. Twitchell, M.D., Clinical Professor of Psychiatry Emeritus.
V. H. Podstata, M.D., Associate Clinical Professor of Psychiatry Emeritus.
Olga Bridgman, M.D., Professor of Psychiatry and Pediatrics.
Paul A. Gliebe, M.D., Assistant Professor of Psychiatry.
D. G. Campbell, M.D., Assistant Clinical Professor of Psychiatry.
J. Kasanin, M.D., Assistant Clinical Professor of Psychiatry.
D. K. Kelley, M.D., Instructor in Psychiatry.
P. P. Poliak, M.D., Clinical Instructor in Psychiatry.
Portia Bell Hume, M.D., Clinical Instructor in Psychiatry.
K. G. Rew, M.D., Clinical Instructor in Psychiatry.
R. M. Ritchey, M.D., Clinical Instructor in Psychiatry.
J. Frostig, M.D., Lecturer and Research Associate in Psychiatry.
Pearl Axelrod, M.S., Lecturer in Psychiatry and Chief Psychiatric Social Worker, the Langley Porter Clinic.
Louise Morrow, M.D., Clinical Instructor in Pediatrics.
Bernard A. Fries, Ph.D., Research Associate in Neurophysiology.
Charles H. Honzik, Ph.D., Research Associate in Psychology.

Institute of Child Welfare, Berkeley

H. E. Jones, Ph.D., Director; Professor of Psychology.
J. W. Macfarlane, Ph.D., Research Associate and Professor of Psychology.
H. S. Conrad, Ph.D., Research Associate and Associate Professor of Psychology.
R. N. Safford, Ph.D., Research Associate and Assistant Professor of Psychology.
H. D. Carter, Ph.D., Research Associate and Assistant Professor of Education.
Anna Espenschade, Ph.D., Research Fellow and Assistant Professor of Physical Education.
Catherine Landreth, Ph.D., Director, Nursery School; Assistant Professor of Home Economics.
P. R. Van Horn, M.D., Research Associate and Assistant Physician.
H. R. Stolz, M.D., Research Associate.
Nancy Bayley, Ph.D., Research Associate.
M. P. Honzik, Ph.D., Research Associate.
N. W. Shock, Ph.D., Research Associate.

E. F. Brunswik, Ph.D., Research Associate.
M. C. Jones, Ph.D., Research Associate.
C. McC. Tryon, Ph.D., Research Associate.
L. M. Stolz, Ph.D., Research Associate.
L. B. Wolff, M.D., Research Associate.
E. H. Erikson, Lecturer and Research Associate.
Lucile Allen, M.A., Nursery School Teacher and Psychologist.
Judith Chaffey, M.A., Research Assistant.
R. D. Tuddenham, Research Assistant.
Wilma Lloyd, M.A., Research Assistant.

CONNECTICUT

Yale University, New Haven

Medical School

Eugen Kahn, M.D., Sterling Professor of Psychiatry and Mental Hygiene.
Edwin F. Gildea, M.D., Associate Professor of Psychiatry and Mental Hygiene.
Lloyd J. Thompson, M.D., Associate Clinical Professor of Psychiatry and Mental Hygiene.
Warren T. Brown, M.D., Assistant Professor of Psychiatry and Mental Hygiene.
Evelyn B. Man, Ph.D., Research Associate in Biochemistry (Assistant Professor).
Walter R. Miles, Ph.D., Professor of Psychology.
Catharine C. Miles, Ph.D., Clinical Professor of Psychology.
Pauline S. Sears, Ph.D., Clinical Instructor of Psychology.

Clinic of Child Development

Arnold Gesell, M.D., Director.
Frances L. Ilg, M.D., Assistant Professor of Child Development.
Henry M. Halverson, Ph.D., Research Associate.
Catherine S. Amatruda, M.D., Research Assistant.
Louise B. Ames, Ph.D., Research Assistant.

DISTRICT OF COLUMBIA

Catholic University of America, Washington

Thomas V. Moore, M.D., Director, Department of Psychology and Psychiatry.
John Russell, M.D., Staff Member.
Gertrude Reiman, Ph.D., M.D., Staff Member.
Katherine Keneally, Research Assistant.

United States Public Health Service, Washington

Public Health Service Hospital, Lexington, Ky.
C. K. Himmelsbach, M.D., Director of Research.
M. J. Pescor, M.D., Clinical Director.
E. G. Williams, M.D., Physiologist and Director of Laboratories.
F. W. Oberst, M.D., Biochemist.
H. L. Andrews, M.D., Biophysicist.
R. R. Brown, Ph.D., Psychologist.

Public Health Service Hospital, Fort Worth, Tex.
W. F. Ossenfort, M.D., Medical Officer in Charge.
Dale C. Cameron, M.D., Executive Officer.
Vernam T. Davis, M.D., Clinical Director.
Nathaniel D. Hirsch, Ph.D., Psychologist.
Wilbur E. Deacon, M.D., Senior Medical Technician.
Murray A. Diamond, M.D., Staff Physician in Charge of Tuberculosis Service.

GEORGIA

University of Georgia School of Medicine and University Hospital, Augusta
Hervey M. Cleckley, M.D., Professor of Neuropsychiatry.
W. F. Hamilton, M.D., Professor of Physiology.
Perry P. Volpitto, M.D., Professor of Anaesthesiology.
R. A. Woodbury, M.D., Associate Professor of Physiology.
Lane Allen, M.D., Associate Professor of Anatomy.
Byrum Beard, M.D., Assistant Resident in Medicine, University Hospital.

ILLINOIS

Institute of General Semantics, Chicago
Alfred Korzybski, Director.
M. Kendig, Educational Director.

Institute for Psychoanalysis, Chicago
Franz Alexander, M.D., Director.
Thomas M. French, M.D., Associate Director.
Catherine L. Bacon, M.D., Member of Clinical Staff.
Therese Benedek, M.D., Member of Clinical Staff.
Margaret W. Gerard, M.D., Member of Clinical Staff.
Martin Grotjahn, M.D., Member of Clinical Staff.
Helen Vincent McLean, M.D., Member of Clinical Staff.
Milton L. Miller, M.D., Member of Clinical Staff.

George J. Mohr, M.D., Member of Clinical Staff.
Leon J. Saul, M.D., Member of Clinical Staff.
Carel Van der Heide, M.D., Member of Clinical Staff.
Ludolf Bollmeier, M.D., Research Associate.
Edwin R. Eisler, M.D., Research Associate.
Rudolf Fuerst, M.D., Research Associate.
Maxwell Gitelson, M.D., Research Associate.
Roy Grinker, M.D., Research Associate.
Adelaid M. Johnson, M.D., Research Associate.
Harry B. Levey, M.D., Research Associate.
Albrecht Meyer, M.D., Research Associate.
Gerhard Piers, M.D., Research Associate.
Helen Ross, Research Associate.
Boris B. Rubenstein, M.D., Research Associate.
Lucie E. Tower, M.D., Research Associate.
Eduardo Weiss, M.D., Research Associate.
George W. Wilson, M.D., Research Associate.

Loyola University and Cook County Hospital, Chicago
John J. Madden, M.D., Chairman of Department.
Francis J. Braceland, M.D., Clinical Professor of Psychiatry.
L. J. Meduna, M.D., Associate Clinical Professor of Psychiatry.
Leo J. Kaplan, M.D., Clinical Associate, Neurology and Psychiatry.
John A. Vaichulis, M.D., Instructor, Department of Physiology.

Michael Reese Hospital, Chicago
Roy R. Grinker, M.D., Chairman of Department.
Maxwell Gitelson, M.D., Director of Psychiatric Services.
Emmy Sylvester, M.D., Associate in Child Psychiatry.
Joseph Reich, M.D., Associate in Neuropsychiatry.
Norman Levy, M.D., Adjunct in Neuropsychiatry.
Eugene Falstein, M.D., Adjunct in Neuropsychiatry.
Winifred Breslin, M.D., Senior Resident.
Joseph Rheingold, M.D., Member of Clinic Staff.
Herman Serota, M.D., Member of Clinic Staff.
Samuel J. Beck, Ph.D., Psychologist.

Northwestern University, Chicago
Lewis J. Pollock, M.D., Professor of Nervous and Mental Diseases.
Clarence A. Neymann, M.D., Associate Professor of Nervous and
Mental Diseases.
Isidore Finkelman, M.D., Assistant Professor of Nervous and
Mental Diseases.
Benjamin Boshes, M.D., Assistant Professor of Nervous and
Mental Diseases.

Alex J. Arieff, M.D., Associate in Department of Nervous and Mental Diseases.

Meyer Brown, M.D., Associate in Department of Nervous and Mental Diseases.

George K. Yacorzynski, M.D., Associate in Department of Nervous and Mental Diseases.

Erich Libert, M.D., Associate in Department of Nervous and Mental Diseases, and Clinical Director, Elgin State Hospital.

Eli L. Tigay, M.D., Instructor in Department of Nervous and Mental Diseases.

Irving C. Sherman, M.D., Instructor in Department of Nervous and Mental Diseases.

University of Chicago, Chicago

Department of Medicine
David Slight, M.D., Professor of Psychiatry.
Hugh T. Carmichael, M.D., Assistant Professor of Psychiatry.
Jules H. Masserman, M.D., Assistant Professor of Psychiatry.
Henry W. Brosin, M.D., Assistant Professor of Psychiatry.
Joan Fleming, M.D., Instructor in Psychiatry.
Adrian VanderVeer, M.D., Instructor in Psychiatry.
Charlotte G. Babcock, M.D., Instructor in Psychiatry.
Anna Elonen, Psychologist.
Martha Johnson, Psychologist.
Ruth Lambert, Psychologist.

Otho S. A. Sprague Memorial Institute
Ward C. Halstead, Ph.D., Assistant Professor in Experimental Psychology.
Theodore J. Case, M.D., Assistant Professor of Neurophysiology.
Eva R. Balken, Ph.D., Instructor in Psychology.
George V. Knox, Ph.D., Research Associate in Experimental Psychology.
Martin Goldner, M.D., Department of Medicine.

Department of Anatomy
Stephen Polyak, M.D., Associate Professor of Anatomy.
David B. Clark, M.D., Research Assistant in Neuroanatomy.

Department of Pharmacology
E. M. K. Geiling, M.D., Professor of Pharmacology.
F. Ellis Kelsey, M.D., Research Associate.

Department of Pathology
Julian H. Lewis, M.D., Associate Professor of Pathology.

Department of Psychology
Heinrich Klüver, Ph.D., Professor of Psychology.

Orthogenic School
Mandel Sherman, M.D., Psychiatrist and Director.
Hudson Jost, Ph.D., Physiological Psychologist and Research Assistant.
Helen Robinson, M.A., Psychologist.

KANSAS

Menninger Sanitarium and Clinic and Southard School, Topeka
C. F. Menninger, M.D., President, Board of Directors.
Karl A. Menninger, M.D., Chief of Staff, The Menninger Clinic.
William C. Menninger, M.D., Medical Director, The Menninger Sanitarium.
Robert P. Knight, M.D., Chief of Psychotherapy Service.
Ernest Lewy, M.D., Senior Staff Member.
Harlan Crank, M.D., Associate Staff Member.
Sylvia Allen, M.D., Associate Staff Member.
Elisabeth Geleerd, M.D., Associate Staff Member.
C. G. Tillman, M.D., Assistant Staff Member.
E. D. Greenwood, M.D., Assistant Staff Member.
Anna Benjamin, M.D., Director, Southard School.
Lewis L. Robbins, M.D., Fellow in Psychiatry.
Merton Gill, M.D., Fellow in Psychiatry.
Milton Layoff, M.D., Resident in Psychiatry.
Mark Stone, M.D., Resident in Psychiatry.
J. F. Brown, Ph.D., Chief, Psychology Department.
David Rapaport, Ph.D., Senior Psychologist.
Margaret Brenman, Junior Psychologist.

KENTUCKY

University of Louisville, Louisville
Spafford Ackerly, M.D., Professor of Psychiatry.
William K. Keller, M.D., Assistant Professor of Psychiatry.
Edw. E. Landis, M.D., Associate in Psychiatry.
Joseph E. Brewer, Ph.D., Psychologist.
Regina Cohn, Psychiatric Social Worker.
Ruth Mellor, Psychiatric Social Worker.

MARYLAND

Chestnut Lodge Sanitarium, Rockville
Dexter M. Bullard, M.D., Physician-in-Charge.

Children's Rehabilitation Institute, Baltimore
Leslie B. Hohman, M.D., Psychiatrist.

Johns Hopkins University, Baltimore

Department of Psychiatry and Henry Phipps Psychiatric Clinic
John C. Whitehorn, M.D., Professor of Psychiatry, Psychiatrist-in-Chief.
Curt P. Richter, M.D., Associate Professor of Psychobiology.
W. Horsley Gantt, M.D., Associate in Psychiatry, Pavlovian Laboratory.
Henry M. Fox, M.D., Associate in Psychiatry.
Alexander H. Leighton, M.D., Instructor in Psychiatry.
Theodore Lidz, M.D., Instructor in Psychiatry.
W. C. Hoffman, M.D., Instructor in Psychiatry.
Katherine Rice, Assistant in Psychobiology.

Children's Psychiatric Service (Harriet Lane Home)
Leo Kanner, M.D., Associate Professor of Psychiatry; Director, Children's Psychiatric Service.
Erich Benjamin, M.D., Research Associate in Psychiatry.
Jacob H. Conn, M.D., Instructor in Psychiatry.
Elizabeth Kane, Assistant in Psychiatry.

School of Hygiene and Public Health
Paul Lemkau, M.D., Psychiatrist; Associate in Public Health Administration.
Christopher Tietze, M.D., Medical Statistician; Research Associate in Mental Hygiene.
Marcia Cooper, M.A., Psychiatric Social Worker.

Department of Medicine
G. Canby Robinson, M.D., Lecturer in Medicine.

Sheppard and Enoch Pratt Hospital, Towson
Ross McC. Chapman, M.D., Superintendent.
Lawrence F. Woolley, M.D., Clinical Director.
T. Douglas Noble, M.D., Senior Physician.
William W. Elgin, M.D., Senior Physician, Chief of Women's Service.

Richard H. Pembroke, Jr., M.D., Resident Physician.
Robert A. Cohen, M.D., Resident Physician.
Allan Burke, M.D., Resident Physician.
Mabel B. Cohen, M.D., Resident Physician.
Jack Jarvis, M.D., Resident Physician.
G. Wilson Shaffer, Ph.D., Psychologist.
Frederick Germuth, Ph.D., Consulting Biological Chemist.
Edward Brown, Pharmacist.
Edna Rose, Technician.
Edward N. Phillips, Technician.

MASSACHUSETTS

Austen Fox Riggs Foundation, Inc., Stockbridge
Charles H. Kimberly, M.D., Medical Director; Research Consultant.
Edgerton McC. Howard, M.D., Director of Research.
Alice F. Raymond, A.B., Associate Research Director.

Beth Israel Hospital, Boston
M. Ralph Kaufman, M.D., Visiting Neuropsychiatrist.
Joseph J. Michaels, M.D., Associate Visiting Neuropsychiatrist.
Samuel H. Epstein, M.D., Junior Visiting Neuropsychiatrist.
Edward Ribring, M.D., Assistant in Neuropsychiatry.
Jennie Waelder, M.D., Assistant in Neuropsychiatry.

Boston City Hospital, Boston
H. Houston Merritt, M. D., Acting Director, Neurological Unit;
    Assistant Professor of Neurology, Harvard Medical School.
William G. Lennox, M.D., Visiting Neurologist; Assistant Professor of Neurology, Harvard Medical School.
Frederic A. Gibbs, M.D., Junior Visiting Neurologist; Instructor, Department of Neurology, Harvard Medical School.
Merrill Moore, M.D., Assistant Visiting Psychiatrist; Associate in Psychiatry, Harvard Medical School.
Charles Brenner, M.D., Assistant to the Visiting Neurologists; Assistant in Neurology, Harvard Medical School.
Wilfred Bloomberg, M.D., Assistant Visiting Neurologist; Instructor in Neurology, Harvard Medical School.
Alexandra Adler, M.D., Assistant to the Visiting Neurologists; Assistant in Neurology, Harvard Medical School.
Raymond D. Adams, M.D., Junior Visiting Neurologist; Instructor in Neurology, Harvard Medical School.
Harry Kozol, M.D., Junior Visiting Neurologist; Instructor in Neurology, Harvard Medical School.

Children's Hospital, Boston
    Bronson Crothers, M.D., Director of Department.
    Randolph K. Byers, M.D., Assistant Director.
    Elizabeth E. Lord, Ph.D., Psychologist.
    Katharine Rickards, Play Supervisor.
    Manon McGinnis, Social Worker.

Habit Clinic for Child Guidance and Tufts College Medical School, Boston
    Douglas A. Thom, M.D., Director.
    Beatrice Schwartz, Research Assistant.

Judge Baker Guidance Center, Boston
    George E. Gardner, M.D., and Frederick Rosenheim, M.D., Directors.
    William Healy, M.D., and Augusta F. Bronner, Ph.D., Consulting Directors.
    Louise Wood, Chief Psychologist.
    Rosamond Clark, Research Assistant.

Massachusetts Department of Mental Health, Boston
    Francis H. Sleeper, M.D., Assistant Commissioner.

Massachusetts General Hospital, Boston
    Stanley Cobb, M.D., Psychiatrist-in-Chief; Bullard Professor of Neuropathology, Harvard Medical School.
    Jacob Ellis Finesinger, M.D., Assistant Professor of Psychiatry, Harvard Medical School.
    Erich Lindemann, M.D., Associate in Psychiatry, Harvard Medical School.
    George Saslow, M.D., Assistant in Psychiatry, Harvard Medical School.
    Mandel E. Cohen, M.D., Instructor in Psychiatry, Harvard Medical School.
    Henry S. Forbes, M.D., Associate in Neuropathology, Harvard Medical School.
    William Chapman, M.D., Wallcott Fellow in Clinical Medicine, Harvard Medical School.
    Robert S. Schwab, M.D., Assistant in Neurology, Harvard Medical School.
    Henry K. Beecher, M.D., Dorr Professor of Research in Anesthesia, Harvard Medical School.
    Elliott D. Chapple, M.D., Research Fellow in Psychiatry.
    Jurgen Ruesch, M.D., Research Fellow in Psychiatry.

McLean Hospital, Waverley
Kenneth J. Tillotson, M.D., Psychiatrist in Charge.

Peter Bent Brigham Hospital, Boston
H. Houston Merritt, M.D., Associate in Medicine; Assistant Professor of Neurology, Harvard Medical School.
Knox Finley, M.D., Junior Associate in Psychiatry; Instructor in Psychiatry, Harvard Medical School.
Roy Swank, M.D., Junior Associate in Medicine; Assistant in Medicine, Harvard Medical School.
George Engel, M.D., Research Fellow, Harvard Medical School.

Supreme Council, 33°, Scottish Rite, Northern Masonic Jurisdiction, Boston
Melvin M. Johnson, Sovereign Grand Commander.
Nolan D. C. Lewis, M.D., Field Representative.

MICHIGAN

Henry Ford Hospital, Detroit
Thomas J. Heldt, M.D., Physician-in-Charge, Division of Neuropsychiatry.
Daniel D. Hurst, M.D., Senior Assistant in Psychiatry.
Laurence D. Trevett, M.D., Senior Assistant in Psychiatry.
Gerald O. Grain, M.D., Associate in Neurology.
Leston S. Whitehead, M.D., Assistant in Psychiatry.
Hawley S. Sanford, M.D., Associate in Psychology.
Emmett L. Schott, Ph.D., Associate in Psychology.
Margaret Ives, Ph.D., Senior Assistant in Psychology.

Wayne University and Eloise Hospital, Detroit
Milton H. Erickson, M.D., Director of Psychiatric Research.

MINNESOTA

University of Minnesota and Minnesota General Hospital, Minneapolis-St. Paul
J. C. McKinley, M.D., Professor of Neuropsychiatry; Head, Department of Medicine; Director, Psychopathic Unit.
A. B. Baker, M.D., Associate Professor of Neuropsychiatry and Neuropathology.
Starke R. Hathaway, Ph.D., Clinical Psychologist; Associate Professor of Psychology.
B. C. Schiele, M.D., Assistant Professor of Neuropsychiatry.

C. G. Polan, M.D., Clinical Assistant in Neuropsychiatry.
L. C. Strough, M.D., Medical Fellow in Neuropsychiatry.
William K. Estes, Teaching Assistant.

MISSOURI

Neurological Hospital, Kansas City
G. Wilse Robinson, M.D., Medical Director.
G. Wilse Robinson, Jr., M.D., Associate Medical Director.
Prioer Shelton, M.D., Staff Psychiatrist.
G. A. Esslinger, M.D., Staff Neurologist and Neuro-surgeon.

Washington University, St. Louis
David McK. Rioch, M.D., Professor of Neurology; Chairman of Department of Neuropsychiatry.
Carlyle F. Jacobsen, M.D., Professor of Medical Psychology.
E. Van Norman Emery, M.D., Professor of Social Psychology and Lecturer in Psychiatry.
Frank J. Bruno, Ph.D., Professor of Applied Sociology.
Samuel R. Warson, M.D., Assistant Professor of Psychiatry.
Andrew B. Jones, Assistant Professor of Clinical Neurology.
Louis L. Tureen, M.D., Assistant Professor of Clinical Neurology.
George H. Bishop, Ph.D., Laboratory of Biophysics.
Herbert J. Erwin, M.D., Resident in Neuropsychiatry, Homer G. Phillips Hospital.
Anthony K. Busch, M.D., Assistant in Clinical Psychiatry.
Henry G. Schwartz, M.D., Instructor in Clinical Neurological Surgery and Neuroanatomy, Department of Surgery.
Leopold Hofstatter, M.D., City Sanitarium.
Irwin Levy, M.D., Instructor in Clinical Neurology.
Hyman H. Fingert, M.D., Instructor in Psychiatry.
William O. Russell, M.D., Instructor in Pathology.
William Reese, B.S., M.S., Student Assistant.
Kent McQueen, B.S., Student Assistant.
Louis Gottschalk, A.B., Student Assistant.

NEBRASKA

University of Nebraska Medical School, Omaha
G. Alexander Young, M.D., Professor of Neuropsychiatry; Chairman of the Department.
A. E. Bennett, M.D., Assistant Professor of Neuropsychiatry.
Richard H. Young, M.D., Assistant Professor of Neuropsychiatry.

Walter Gysin, M.D., Resident Psychiatrist, Douglas County Hospital.

Paul Cash, M.D., Instructor in Neuropsychiatry.

Avis B. Purdy, R.N., Psychiatric Supervisor.

June McLeod, Nursing Supervisor in Fever Therapy.

NEW JERSEY

Training School at Vineland

Edgar A. Doll, Ph.D., Director of Reseaarch.

H. Robert Otness, Ph.D., Chief Clinician.

Kathryn F. Deacon, A.B., Research Assistant.

NEW YORK

Albany Hospital and Albany Medical College, Albany

D. Ewen Cameron, M.D., Psychiatrist and Neurologist-in-Chief.

J. D. Sullivan, M.D., Resident in Neurology and Psychiatry.

H. Aldendorff, M.D., Assistant Resident in Neurology and Psychiatry.

H. Himwich, Ph.D., Professor of Psychology.

F. Feldman, Student Research Assistant.

Committee for the Study of Sex Variants, New York

George W. Henry, M.D., Psychiatrist.

Alfred A. Gross, Research Assistant.

Hillside Hospital, New York

Louis Wender, M.D., Medical Director.

Erwin Levy, M.D., Senior Psychiatrist.

Abraham Jezer, M.D., Consultant Cardiologist.

Jewish Board of Guardians, New York

Richard L. Frank, M.D., Psychiatrist.

J. H. N. Van Ophuijsen, M.D., Psychiatrist.

Frederika Neumann, Case Consultant.

Ruth Eastwood Perl, Ph.D., Statistician.

Irving Ryckoff, Case Worker.

Lifwynn Foundation, New York

Trigant Burrow, M.D., Ph.D., Scientific Director.

Clarence Shields, A.B., Research Associate.

Hans Syz, M.D., Research Associate.
Charles B. Thompson, M.D., Research Assistant.
William Galt, M.A., Ph.D., Research Assistant.

Mount Sinai Hospital, New York
Department of Neurology—Psychiatric Division
Israel S. Wechsler, M.D., Neurologist.
Laurence S. Kubie, M.D., Associate Psychiatrist.
Sidney Margolin, M.D., Research Fellow.
Sol Ginsburg, M.D., Adjunct.
Rene A. Spitz, M.D., Adjunct.
Eric Morse, M.D., Clinical Assistant.
Isador Silberman, M.D., Clinical Assistant.
Emil A. Gutheil, M.D., Clinical Assistant.
P. Goolker, M.D., Clinical Assistant.
Edgar Trautman, M.D., Clinical Assistant.
Edith Klemperer, M.D., Clinical Assistant.
Mark Kanzer, M.D., Clinical Assistant.
Sidney Tarachow, M.D., Clinical Assistant.
Samuel Atkin, M.D., Research Assistant.
Eugene C. Milch, M.D., Research Assistant.

Department of Pediatrics—Children's Health Class
Ira S. Wile, M.D., Associate in Pediatrics.
Richard Frank, M.D., Assistant in Pediatrics.
Carl Pototsky, M.D., Assistant in Pediatrics.
Rose Davis, Psychologist.

New York Hospital—Cornell University Medical Center, New York
Payne Whitney Psychiatric Clinic
Oskar Diethelm, M.D., Professor of Psychiatry.
Thomas A. C. Rennie, M.D., Associate Professor of Psychiatry.
Harold G. Wolff, M.D., Associate Professor of Medicine (Neurology).
Ade T. Milhorat, M.D., Assistant Professor of Medicine.
Milton J. E. Senn, M.D., Assistant Professor of Pediatrics.
J. Louise Despert, M.D., Research Associate in Psychiatry.
Edwin J. Doty, M.D., Instructor in Psychiatry.
Francis J. Hamilton, M.D., Instructor in Psychiatry.
Marianne Horney, M.D., Instructor in Psychiatry.
Herbert S. Ripley, M.D., Instructor in Psychiatry.
Fred V. Rockwell, M.D., Instructor in Psychiatry.
Saul M. Small, M.D., Instructor in Psychiatry.
Marshall R. Jones, Instructor in Psychology.
Donald J. Simons, M.D., Instructor in Medicine.

Westchester Division, White Plains
Clarence O. Cheney, M.D., Medical Director.
James H. Wall, M.D., Assistant Medical Director.
Hollis E. Clow, M.D., Director of Laboratories and Resident Internist.
Donald M. Hamilton, M.D., Resident Physician.
Jean Blauvelt, Psychologist.

New York Infirmary for Women and Children, New York
Margaret E. Fries, M.D., Director of Studies; Consultant to Pediatric Service.
Beatrice Lewi, Assistant to Director.
Leona Levine, B.S., Psychologist.
Grace Green, B.S., Psychologist.
Paul J. Woolf, B.S., Photographer.
Frances Gmelch, R.N., Superintendent of Nurses.
Evelyn Downing, B.S., R.N., Supervisor of Clinics.
Bela Schick, M.D., Consultant Pediatrician.

New York Post Graduate Hospital and Medical School, New York
Philip R. Lehrman, M.D., Attending Neurologist and Psychiatrist; Clinical Professor of Neurology and Psychiatry, Columbia University.
Sidney Klein, M.D., Associate Attending Neurologist and Psychiatrist; Assistant Clinical Professor of Neurology and Psychiatry, Columbia University.
Alexander D. Tendler, Ph.D., Attending Psychologist.
Harry M. Shulman, Ph.B., Attending Psychologist, Dispensary Service.
Helen Thompson, Ph.D., Associate Attending Psychologist, Dispensary Service.
Arnold Eisendorfer, M.D., Assistant Attending Neurologist and Psychiatrist.
Ruth Loveland, M.D., Assistant Attending Neurologist and Psychiatrist.
Frances Cottington, M.D., Assistant Attending Neurologist and Psychiatrist, Dispensary Service.

New York State Department of Mental Hygiene, Albany
Horatio M. Pollock, Ph.D., Director, Bureau of Statistics.
Benjamin Malzberg, Ph.D., Senior Statistician.

New York Vocational Adjustment Bureau for Girls, New York
Emily T. Burr, Ph.D., Director.
Harriet Babcock, Ph.D., Psychologist.

(Mrs.) Zaida Metcalfe, Placement Counselor and Research Worker.
Hedwig Jahoda, Ph.D., Volunteer.

Pinewood, Katonah

Joseph Epstein, M.D., Director.
Max Friedemann, M.D., Associate Physician.
Barnett Rosenblum, M.D., Associate Physician.

Stony Lodge, Ossining

Bernard Glueck, M.D., Medical Director.
Josephine S. Glueck, M.D., Assistant Medical Director.
Emy A. Metzger, M.D., Resident Physician.
Leon L. Altman, M.D., Resident Physician.
Hilde Koppel, M.D., Interne.
Dallas Pratt, Interne.

Syracuse Psychopathic Hospital and Syracuse University, Syracuse

Harry A. Steckel, M.D., Director.
Eugene Davidoff, M.D., Senior Clinical Psychiatrist.
Gerald L. Goodstone, M.D., Resident Physician.
E. C. Reifenstein, Jr., M.D., Clinic Physician.
Albert B. Siewers, M.D., Clinic Physician.
Noble R. Chambers, M.D., Clinic Physician.
Elinor S. Noetzel, Senior Psychiatric Social Worker.
Gertrude Buckland, Volunteer Speech, Reading and Dramatic Teacher.
Susan Stabile, Volunteer Music Teacher.
Frances Nicoll, Chief Occupational Therapist.
Sarah McLean, Occupational Therapist.

OHIO

University of Cincinnati and Cincinnati General Hospital, Cincinnati

Department of Anatomy
Edward F. Malone, M.D., Professor of Anatomy.
Lawrence O. Morgan, Ph.D., Associate Professor of Anatomy.
A. R. Vonderahe, M.D., Associate Professor of Anatomy.
William Niemer, Research Associate in Anatomy.

Department of Physiology
Gustav Eckstein, D.D.S., M.D., L.H.D., Associate Professor of Physiology.
Howard Fabing, M.D., Instructor in Physiology; Assistant Attending Neurologist, Neurologic Division, Department of Medicine.

Department of Biochemistry
Shiro Tashiro, Ph.D., Professor of Biochemistry.
Elizabeth Badger, Research Assistant.
Kazu Tashiro, Research Assistant.
Carl Schmidt, Ph.D., Research Assistant.

Department of Pharmacology
Dennis Emerson Jackson, Ph.D., M.D., Professor of Pharmacology.

Department of Psychology
Arthur G. Bills, Ph.D., Professor of Psychology.
E. L. Talbert, Ph.D., Associate Professor of Psychology.
Virginia Graham, Ph.D., Lecturer in Clinical Psychology.
William Griffith, Research Assistant.

Department of Psychiatry
John Romano, M.D., Professor of Psychiatry; Director, Department of Psychiatry, Cincinnati General Hospital.
Othilda Krug Brady, M.D., M.S., Resident in Psychiatry, Cincinnati General Hospital.

Laboratory of Neuropathology
Charles D. Aring, M.D., Associate Professor of Neurology.
Thomas Douglas Spies, M.D., Associate Professor of Medicine.
Eugene B. Ferris, M.D., Assistant Professor of Medicine.
Milton Rosenbaum, M.D., Assistant Professor of Psychiatry.
Henry W. Ryder, M.D., Instructor in Medicine.
George Maltby, M.D., Research Associate.

May Institute for Medical Research
Arthur Mirsky, M.D., Director.
David L. Abramson, M.D., Associate, in charge of Cardiovascular Research.
Alfred Frolich, M.D., Associate, in charge of Pharmacological Studies.
Samuel Elgart, M.D., Research Fellow.

Child Guidance Home
Louis A. Lurie, M.D., Director; Assistant Professor of Psychiatry.
Jack Hertzman, M.D., Attending Psychiatrist.
Sol Levy, M.D., Resident Physician.
(Mrs.) Dudley Miller Outcalt, Psychologist.
(Mrs.) William H. Rosenthal, Director of Psychiatric Social Service.
(Mrs.) Osna B. Lurie, Social Worker.

Children's Hospital
Albert B. Sabin, M.D., Director.
Robert Ward, M.D., Assistant Professor of Pediatrics.

Carl E. Duffy, Ph.D., Research Assistant.
Joel Warren, Ph.D., Research Assistant.
Isaac Ruchman, M.S., Research Assistant.

Longview Hospital

Douglas Goldman, M.D., Clinical Director.
Francis Marion Stephens, M.D., Resident Physician.
Lucille Limbach, M.D., Resident Physician.
Norman Schkloven, M.D., Resident Physician; Assistant, Department of Psychiatry.
Sanford Birnbaum, M.S., Department of Biochemistry.
Evelyn Partymiller, M.D., Assistant Physician.
Werner Hollander, M.D., Assistant Physician.
Else Weyman, M.D., Assistant Physician.

Western Reserve University, Cleveland

City Hospital

Louis J. Karnosh, M.D., Resident Director, Psychopathic Division, City Hospital.
Edward Zucker, M.D., Chief Resident in Neuropsychiatry.
Alan Adam, M.D., Resident in Neuropsychiatry.
Harry Lipson, M.D., Junior Visitant, Department of Neuropsychiatry.

Cleveland Guidance Center

Henry C. Schumacher, M.D., Director.

OREGON

University of Oregon Medical School, Portland

Henry H. Dixon, M.D., Clinical Professor of Psychiatry.
John C. Evans, M.D., Assistant Clinical Professor of Psychiatry; Superintendent, Salem State Hospital.
D. C. Burkes, M.D., Clinical Associate.
W. H. Hutchens, M.D., Medical Associate.
G. B. Haugen, M.D., Medical Associate.
John L. Haskins, M.D., Clinical Instructor; Superintendent, Morningside Hospital.
John W. Evans, M.D., Medical Instructor.
Lewis C. Martin, Ph.D., Psychologist.
Allan W. East, M.A., Supervisor of Social Work, State Child Guidance Clinic Extension.
Gladys Dobson, M.S., Supervisor of Visiting Teachers, Portland Child Guidance Clinic.

PENNSYLVANIA

Elwyn Training School, Elwyn
E. A. Whitney, M.D., Superintendent.
Joseph E. Nowrey, M.D., Senior Assistant Physician.

Gladwyne Colony, Gladwyne
S. De W. Ludlum, M.D., Director, Gladwyne Research Laboratory.

Jefferson Medical College, Philadelphia
Baldwin L. Keyes, M.D., Professor of Psychiatry.

Philadelphia Child Guidance Clinic, Philadelphia
Frederick H. Allen, M.D., Director.
Miss Almena Dawley, Chief Psychiatric Social Worker.
Miss Marion Nicholson, Psychiatric Social Worker.
Miss Dorothy Hankins, Psychiatric Social Worker.

Philadelphia General Hospital, Philadelphia
Annie E. Taft, M.D., Research Associate, Psychiatric Department.
Helena E. Riggs, M.D., Pathologist to Psychiatric Department.

Temple University School of Medicine, Philadelphia
Ernest A. Spiegel, M.D., Professor of Experimental Neurology.
Mona Spiegel-Adolf, M.D., Professor of Colloidal Chemistry.
O. Spurgeon English, M.D., Clinical Professor of Psychiatry.
Herbert Freed, M.D., Instructor in Psychiatry.
(Mrs.) June B. Read, Research Assistant.
Morton J. Oppenheimer, M.D., Associate Professor of Physiology.
Henry T. Wycis, M.D., Resident in Neurosurgery.
Norman P. Scala, M.D., Instructor in Ophthalmology, Georgetown
    University, Washington, D. C.
G. C. Hennie, M.D., Director, Department of Physics.

University of Pennsylvania—Pennsylvania Hospital, Philadelphia
Lauren H. Smith, M.D., Physician-in-Chief and Administrator
Earl D. Bond, M.D., Director of Research.
Edward A. Strecker, M.D., Consultant-in-Chief.
Bernard J. Alpers, M.D., Neuropathologist and Consultant.
Joseph Hughes, M.D., Director of Laboratories.
Edward M. Westburgh, Ph.D., Chief of Psychological Service.
Donald Hastings, M.D., Psychiatrist.
Thurston Rivers, M.D., Psychiatrist.
Louis Twyeffort, M.D., Psychiatrist.

Howard Rome, M.D., Psychiatrist.
David Wright, M.D., Psychiatrist.
John Appel, M.D., Psychiatrist.
Robert Wigton, M.D., Psychiatrist.
James A. Flaherty, M.D., Psychiatrist.
Detlev W. Bronk, Ph.D., Department of Neurophysiology.
Carl F. Schmidt, Ph.D., Department of Neurophysiology.

RHODE ISLAND

Butler Hospital, Providence
Arthur H. Ruggles, M.D., Superintendent.
George Harold Alexander, M.D., Clinical Director.
Ira C. Nichols, M.D., Physician in Charge of Male Services.
J. McVicker Hunt, Ph.D., Department of Psychology, Brown
University.

Emma Pendleton Bradley Home, East Providence
Charles Bradley, M.D., Superintendent.
Donald B. Lindsley, Ph.D., Director, Psychology Department.
Gertrud Müller, M.D., Resident Physician.
Margaret Bowen, R.N., Research Assistant.

TENNESSEE

Vanderbilt University School of Medicine, Nashville
Frank H. Luton, M.D., Associate Professor of Psychiatry.
William F. Roth, Jr., M.D., Director, Williamson County Child
Guidance Study (State Department of Public Health).
William F. Orr, Jr., M.D., Assistant in Neurology and Psychiatry.
Thomas Butler, M.D., Assistant Professor of Pharmacology.
Virginia Kirk, Field Worker.
(Mrs.) Phyliss Dunham, Field Worker.
Elizabeth Neubert, Field Worker.

VIRGINIA

Tucker Hospital, Richmond
Beverley R. Tucker, M.D., Chief of Staff; Emeritus Professor of
Neuropsychiatry, Medical College of Virginia.
Howard R. Masters, M.D., Associate Chief of Staff; Associate
Professor of Neuropsychiatry, Medical College of Virginia.

James Asa Shield, M.D., Associate Chief of Staff; Associate in Neuropsychiatry, Medical College of Virginia.

Harry Brick, M.D., Resident Physician; Instructor in Neuropsychiatry, Medical College of Virginia.

Westbrook Sanatorium, Richmond
James K. Hall, Medical Superintendent.

WISCONSIN

Milwaukee Sanitarium, Wauwatosa
Lloyd H. Ziegler, M.D., Associate Medical Director.
Merle Q. Howard, M.D., Staff Member.
Carroll W. Osgood, M.D., Staff Member.
Benjamin Ruskin, M.D., Staff Member.
Stuart McWhorter, M.D., Resident

APPENDIX " C "

Sources and Extent of Financial Support for Current Researches

CALIFORNIA

California Department of Institutions, Sacramento

Rosenberg Foundation, California Institute of Technology, and Department of Institutions share in support of researches in shock therapies.

Mount Zion Hospital, San Francisco

No exact allocation of funds. Investigations are financed from hospital budget on approval of research committee.

Stanford University, San Francisco

Erwin Foundation contributes $5,000 for studies in epilepsy; $3,000 received from a private donor for research in pain; $1,500 received from Wine Growers' Association for studies in alcohol; and $1,500 contributed by the university for medical research.

University of California, San Francisco

Medical Center
(Information not available.)

Institute of Child Welfare, Berkeley
Established in 1927 under a grant from Laura Spelman Rockefeller Fund, with supplementary assistance from California Parent-Teacher Association. Since 1935, maintained by University of California, with grants for special research made from time to time by Rockefeller Foundation and General Education Board. Work has also been conducted under a grant-in-aid to the director of the Institute from Social Science Research Council, and under a series of fellowships from Bivin Foundation.

CONNECTICUT

Yale University, New Haven

Psychiatric department at present financed by Rockefeller Foundation; current researches almost exclusively supported from this

191

source. Clinic of Child Development supported by Yale University and by grants from Rockefeller Foundation and Carnegie Corporation.

DISTRICT OF COLUMBIA

Catholic University of America, Washington
Research in department of psychiatry financed from departmental budget, plus $1,800 grant from Rockefeller Foundation. A small budget is provided by the university for clinical expenses at the Child Center, and an additional budget of $570 is available for the department of psychology.

United States Public Health Service, Washington
Researches financed from regular departmental appropriations.

GEORGIA

University of Georgia School of Medicine and University Hospital, Augusta
No special funds available for research.

ILLINOIS

Institute of General Semantics, Chicago
No special funds for research. Financed from general budget.

Institute for Psychoanalysis, Chicago
Research supported by a grant from Rockefeller Foundation, by contributions from individuals, and by income from tuition and patients' fees. A grant also received recently from Mary W. Harriman Trust Fund for special work.

Loyola University and Cook County Hospital, Chicago
Research work supported entirely by university funds. Approximately $10,000 expended to date.

Michael Reese Hospital, Chicago
Research activities supported entirely by funds obtained from endowments and yearly grants disbursed by the research committee of the hospital.

Northwestern University, Chicago

Major sources of financial support for research derived from regular appropriations for the department of nervous and mental diseases under medical school budget. Certain projects related to national defense subsidized in part by Federal funds obtained through National Research Council.

University of Chicago, Chicago

Research activities of division of psychiatry supported by Rockefeller Foundation and Otho S. A. Sprague Memorial Institute. Other projects related to psychiatry conducted in other university departments under funds from Sprague Memorial Institute. Total appropriation for the year 1941-42: $90,734. Breakdown of teaching and research costs not available. Annual grant of $1,000 from Supreme Council, 33°, Northern Masonic Jurisdiction, U.S.A., for studies in dementia praecox. About $5,000 appropriated annually for research at Orthogenic School by University of Chicago.

KANSAS

Menninger Sanitarium and Clinic and Southard School, Topeka

Funds for research derived from Menninger Foundation and other sources. Grants from Menninger Foundation for ten-year study of the place of occupational therapy in psychiatric treatment, for research in the use of hypnosis in emergency psychotherapy and in substantiating newer psychiatric theories, and for other activities.

KENTUCKY

University of Louisville, Louisville

Grant of $50,000 from Commonwealth Fund for experimental program for development of teaching methods in psychiatry for undergraduate medical students and interns (research in methodology). Younger Woman's Club of Louisville contributes $2,100 ($700 a year for three years) for experimental nursery school. Bivin Foundation contributed $200 for follow-up study of children in nursery school; also $500 from the same source for experimental seminars for kindergarten and first-grade teachers in public schools. Private donations help in carrying out electroencephalographic studies. All other clinic researches carried on without special appropriations.

MARYLAND

Chestnut Lodge ·Sanitarium, Rockville
Funds for research derived entirely from current hospital revenue.

Children's Rehabilitation Institute, Baltimore
No special funds set aside for research.

Johns Hopkins University, Baltimore
Annual grants as follows: $12,745 from Rockefeller Foundation for psychobiological laboratory; $3,900 from John and Mary R. Markle Foundation for skin resistance study; $2,800 from Research Council on Problems of Alcohol for alcohol work; $6,000 from Corn Industries Research Fund for food studies; $2,100 from National Research Council for study of cyclical changes; $10,105 from Rockefeller Foundation for Pavlovian laboratory; $5,040 from Epilepsy Medical Research Fund for research in epilepsy and electroencephalography; $3,000 from Supreme Council, 33°, Northern Masonic Jurisdiction, U.S.A., for studies in dementia praecox; $1,732, anonymous, for research in psychiatry and catatonia fund; $3,780 from John and Mary R. Markle Foundation for analysis of case records; $13,800 from Rockefeller Foundation for studies in child psychiatry; and $12,000 from Rockefeller Foundation for mental hygiene study in Eastern Health District.

Sheppard and Enoch Pratt Hospital, Towson
All research activities financed from hospital income.

MASSACHUSETTS

Austen Fox Riggs Foundation, Inc., Stockbridge
Researches into the psychoneuroses, recently completed, sponsored by the John and Mary R. Markle Foundation. Study of psychiatric services in New England colleges, current project, supported by donations from former patients.

Beth Israel Hospital, Boston
Psychiatric research activities supported for the most part by Associated Jewish Philanthropies. No financial aid from any other source.

Boston City Hospital, Boston
Research in epilepsy, requiring about $25,000 annually, financed mostly by special grants from various Foundations, by a pharma-

ceutical firm, and by popular subscriptions to Harvard Epilepsy Commission.

Children's Hospital, Boston

Harvard Medical School contributes toward professional salaries. Children's Hospital supports social service activities. Grants from Commonwealth Fund and Earhart Foundation.

Habit Clinic for Child Guidance and Tufts College Medical School, Boston

Research activities are a by-product of routine clinic work. About half of clinic time of the director devoted to research, plus one research worker on part-time, equivalent to a total of approximately $4,000; financed largely from clinic budget, plus small amount from special fund.

Judge Baker Guidance Center, Boston

Regular budget of the center provides for proportion of research time and assistance for the clinical staff. Funds for research on half-time by the co-directors have for several years been given equally by two donors.

Massachusetts Department of Mental Health, Boston

Grants for special statistical studies received from Laura Spelman Rockefeller Fund and Rockefeller Foundation in 1928, 1931 and 1935. Project ended October 1, 1941.

Massachusetts General Hospital, Boston

(Normal research activities suspended with onset of war. Superseded by research project in military psychiatry undertaken for National Research Council.)

McLean Hospital, Waverley

(Information not available.)

Peter Bent Brigham Hospital, Boston

Grant received from Commonwealth Fund in 1941, for two- to three-year period, for teaching, clinical and investigative activities. Sum of $7,900 made available from this source in 1941. In addition, $1,500 appropriated annually by Harrington Fund, for psychological testing.

Supreme Council, 33°, Scottish Rite, Northern Masonic Jurisdiction, Boston

(See Chapter VII, pages 104–107.)

MICHIGAN

Henry Ford Hospital, Detroit
No special research funds. Investigations are conducted by department staff members incidental to clinical work and are covered by department's maintenance budget.

Wayne University and Eloise Hospital, Detroit
No specific grants. Research work supported under county appropriations to Eloise Hospital for institutional maintenance.

MINNESOTA

University of Minnesota and Minnesota General Hospital, Minneapolis-St. Paul
Varying amounts, totalling $8,825, available for research from various sources, including Works Progress Administration, National Youth Administration, Graduate School of the University of Minnesota, and Department of Medicine budget for supplies.

MISSOURI

Neurological Hospital, Kansas City
Research work financed largely from patients' fees. About $750 received from various drug firms for special activities.

Washington University, St. Louis
Most psychiatric research at this center financed from the regular budget of the department, which receives $50,000 a year from Rockefeller Foundation. Of this, about $12,000 is for research. In addition, $3,700 for two years received from Josiah Macy, Jr., Foundation, plus $2,500 from Julius Rosenwald Fund. Also $2,000 from Supreme Council, 33°, Northern Masonic Jurisdiction, U.S.A.

NEBRASKA

University of Nebraska Medical School, Omaha
Research supported from private endowment and by fever therapy research department.

NEW JERSEY

Training School at Vineland
During 1941, approximately $10,000 allocated to research from institution's Maintenance Fund, plus $3,900 in donations from Five Year Plan fund, and $3,100 in interest from Child Study Foundation.

NEW YORK

Albany Hospital and Albany Medical College, Albany
Researches financed entirely from hospital and medical school funds.

Committee for the Study of Sex Variants, New York
(Information not available.)

Hillside Hospital, New York
Research financed at present as part of running expenses of institution.

Jewish Board of Guardians, New York
Two current projects supported by private contributions totalling $8,000; other studies financed from organization's operating budget.

Lifwynn Foundation, New York
Researches financed through Foundation's income, which consists largely of contributions from its scientific staff and working members, plus small endowment for accessories.

Mount Sinai Hospital, New York
Abrahamson Research Fellowship of $2,000 and Kastor Research Fellowship of $1,000 available to department of neurology—psychiatric division; plus small grants from Josiah Macy, Jr., Foundation for research in psychosomatic medicine in department of neurology. No special funds for psychiatric research in pediatric department, except grant from Max J. Breitenbach Fund for services of psychologist.

New York Hospital—Cornell University Medical Center, New York

Payne Whitney Psychiatric Clinic
Research work currently supported by funds from the department of psychiatry (Payne Whitney Psychiatric Clinic). During

academic year 1940–41 additional support received from Commonwealth Fund and Littauer Foundation.

Westchester Division, White Plains
Sole source of income for research at present is Consultation Fee Fund, a fund in which all fees from consultations by all staff members are pooled.

New York Infirmary for Women and Children, New York
Except for temporary support by Works Progress Administration, through. assignment of personnel, researches have been financed from private contributions, including a special fund of $3,000, an annual donation of $600 over a four-year period, and approximately $8,000 contributed by investigator in charge of program.

New York Post Graduate Hospital and Medical School, New York
Present researches financed by Neurological and Psychiatric Fund of approximately $1,500; supplemented by contributions from members of faculty representing their share of teaching honoraria.

New York State Department of Mental Hygiene, Albany
Statistical studies financed from regular department budget, supplemented by funds of Temporary Commission on State Hospital Problems.

New York Vocational Adjustment Bureau for Girls, New York
Studies financed from operating budget of organization, which has been supported by private funds, grants from Greater New York Fund, Federation for the Support of Jewish Philanthropic Societies, foundations and memberships.

Pinewood, Katonah
Research activities supported from earnings or capital funds of institution.

Stony Lodge, Ossining
Research activities supported from hospital earnings.

Syracuse Psychopathic Hospital and Syracuse University, Syracuse
Grant of $1,400 from Smith, Kline & French Laboratories, Philadelphia, Pa., to Syracuse University College of Medicine and E. C. Riefenstein, Jr., M.D., for research in amphetamine sulfate. Grant of $200 from Hendricks Fund of Syracuse University College of Medicine to Gertrude S. Buckland for study of reading disabilities in children.

OHIO

University of Cincinnati and Cincinnati General Hospital, Cincinnati
An undetermined amount of research time covered by departmental budgets of the medical school and by State appropriations to Longview Hospital. Grant of $1,500 a year for several years available for special work from Supreme Council, 33°, Northern Masonic Jurisdiction, U.S.A. A proportion of expense for research at Child Guidance Home defrayed from private funds. May Institute for Medical Research finances a series of studies by its workers.

Western Reserve University, Cleveland

City Hospital
No regular income for research. Investigations conducted incidental to clinical routine. During 1940 and 1941, sum of $1,000 received each year from anonymous donor to purchase special research equipment.

Cleveland Guidance Center
No special funds for research.

OREGON

University of Oregon Medical School, Portland
No special funds for research.

PENNSYLVANIA

Elwyn Training School, Elwyn
No special funds for research.

Gladwyne Colony, Gladwyne
Researches supported from funds of the sanitarium to the amount of $5,000 yearly.

Jefferson Medical College, Philadelphia
No special funds for research.

Philadelphia Child Guidance Clinic, Philadelphia
No special funds for research.

Philadelphia General Hospital, Philadelphia
Researches financed in part from John C. Dawson Fund and from private funds.

Temple University School of Medicine, Philadelphia
Except for occasional grants received in the past from American Medical Association and other sources, no special research funds now available.

University of Pennsylvania—Pennsylvania Hospital, Philadelphia
Approximately $10,000 at present available to Pennsylvania Hospital for research and approximately $15,000 for psychiatric training. Sources of support: Rockefeller Foundation, John and Mary R. Markle Foundation, New York Foundation, and Supreme Council, 33°, Northern Masonic Jurisdiction, U.S.A.

RHODE ISLAND

Butler Hospital, Providence
Received $1,000 from outside sources in 1941 for research studies.

Emma Pendleton Bradley Home, East Providence
Clinical studies in electroencephalography supported until recently by Rockefeller Foundation. Clinical studies of schizophrenia in childhood supported by annual grant of $1,350 from Supreme Council, 33°, Northern Masonic Jurisdiction, U.S.A.

TENNESSEE

Vanderbilt University School of Medicine, Nashville
Williamson County study financed entirely by Rockefeller Foundation for past six years under grant of $16,000 per year to the state health department. Limited financing for research in the general field of narcosis through contributions from a pharmaceutical firm to the university's department of pharmacology.

VIRGINIA

Tucker Hospital, Richmond
During 1940–41, $2,400 available under a fellowship grant from Nemours Foundation.

Westbrook Sanatorium, Richmond
Studies financed from sanatorium income.

WISCONSIN

Milwaukee Sanitarium, Wauwatosa
No special research grants. Research time, materials and supplies covered by regular institutional income.

BIBLIOGRAPHY

SELECTED REFERENCES

AMERICAN ASSOCIATION FOR THE ADVANCEMENT OF SCIENCE. Mental Health. (Section II—Orientation and Methods in Psychiatric Research). Science Press, 1939.

BOND, E. D. Balance in psychiatric research. *Journal of Nervous and Mental Disease.* 89:419–22, April, 1939.

DAYTON, NEIL. Research workers, every one. *Proceedings, American Association on Mental Deficiency.* 44:16–32, 1939 (No. 1).

DOLL, EDGAR A. The meaning of research. *Bulletin of the Training School at Vineland, N. J.* Pp. 181–186, January, 1940.

EBAUGH, F. G. and RYMER, C. A. Teaching and research in state hospitals. *American Journal of Psychiatry.* 96:535–49, November, 1939.

GREGG, ALAN. Furtherance of medical research. Yale University Press, 1941.

————. The significance of research in mental disorders. *Mental Hygiene.* 23:1–11, January, 1939.

KASANIN, JACOB. The problem of research in mental hospitals. *American Journal of Psychiatry.* 92:397–405, September, 1935.

LEWIS, NOLAN D. C. The pluristic approach to psychiatric research. *1940 Yearbook of Neurology, Psychiatry and Endocrinology.* Pp. 319–28, 1941.

————. Research in dementia praecox (past attainments, present trends and future possibilities). The National Committee for Mental Hygiene, 1936.

————. A short history of psychiatric achievement. Norton, 1941.

THE NATIONAL COMMITTEE FOR MENTAL HYGIENE. Research in mental hospitals. The National Committee for Mental Hygiene, 1938.

NATIONAL RESEARCH COUNCIL. Committee on psychiatric investigations. Problem of mental disorder. McGraw, 1934.

NATIONAL RESOURCES COMMITTEE—SCIENCE COMMITTEE. Research—a national resource. I. Relation of the federal government to research. Superintendent of Documents, 1938.

REVIEW OF PSYCHIATRIC PROGRESS, 1941. *American Journal of Psychiatry.* 98:581–603, January, 1942.

SINGER, H. DOUGLAS. Research in psychiatry. *Journal of the American Medical Association.* 104:223–26, June 22, 1935.

THE SUPPORT OF PSYCHIATRIC RESEARCH AND TEACHING. *Psychiatry.* 2:273–79, May, 1939.

WHITEHORN, J. C. and ZILBOORG, GREGORY. Present trends in American psychiatric research. *American Journal of Psychiatry.* 13:303–12, September, 1933.

YEARBOOK OF NEUROLOGY, PSYCHIATRY AND ENDOCRINOLOGY. 4 Vols., 1938–1941. Chicago, Yearbook Publishers, 1939–1942.

ZILBOORG, GREGORY AND HENRY, GEORGE W. A History of Medical Psychology. Norton, 1941.

INDEX

(References are to pages.)

A

Abilities, potential, scientific determination of, 119
Acetone, 122
Acetylcholine, 120
Achievement, psychometric studies of, 117
Achlorhydria, 124
Addison's disease, 44
Adjusted and maladjusted persons, differentiation of, 129
Adjustment, religion as a factor in, 35
Administrative research, 103, 104
Admission studies, 76, 79
Adolescence, relationship to early childhood, 117
Adolescent girls, group treatment of, 126
Adolescents, The Growth Study of, 98
Adoption, 56, 80
Adrenal balance in blood, 107
Adrenal-ectomized cases, 51
Adult-child relationships, institutes on problems of, 128
Affect, role of frontal lobe in, 91
Affectional capacity, deficiencies in, 58
Age
  relationship to dysrhythmia, 53
  cerebral changes in ageing, 75
Age-problem relations, 46
Albany, N. Y., research projects, 25–26, 101–2
Albany Hospital and Albany Medical College, Albany
  report of research projects, 25–26
  list of current research projects, 159
  research personnel, 181
  financial support, 197
Albinism, 124
Albumin, determination of, 87

Alcohol
  reactions to, 44
  in blood stream, 73
Alcoholic patients, therapy of, 37
Alcoholism, 96, 111
  development of therapy, 54
  clinical and laboratory aspects, 72
  physiological changes, 94
  correlation with pellagra, 124
  psychoanalytic studies of, 129
Alhambra Sanatorium, Rosemead, Cal., 99
Allergies, 91
American Medical Association, census of hospitals, 1
American Otological Society laboratory, 27
American Psychiatric Association, 144
Analgesics, 109
Anatomy
  relative to study of loss of weight, 35
  facilities for research in, 70
Anker Hospital, St. Paul, Minn., 31
Anger, 139
Animal experimentation, 86, 89, 99
  facilities for, 25, 34, 44, 53, 63, 67
  relative to study of loss of weight, 35
  effects of cerebral anoxia experimentally induced, 66
  "experimental neuroses" in animals, 91
Animals
  studies of, 30
  elimination of "neurosis," 44
  neuropathological manifestations, 44–45
Anorexia nervosa, 35, 57
Anthropological conditions, 139
Anthropological studies, 107, 118
Anticonvulsants, 94

205

Consultation service, 25, 26, 43, 45, 46, 47, 52, 54, 67, 79, 82, 126, 127, 134
Convalescence, 65
Convalescent home, 54
Convulsions, 37, 88
relation to mental deficiency and retardation, 56
studies of, 73
Convulsive disorders
relationship with dysrhythmia, 53
research at Boston Habit Clinic, 56
permeability of brain cells in, 89
spinal fluid in, 89
influence of drugs, 121
Cook County (Ill.) Criminal Court, Psychopathic Laboratory, 63
Cook County (Ill.) Psychopathic Hospital, 59, 61, 63, 67, 149, 173, 192
Cornell University Medical College, 114
See also New York Hospital-Cornell University Medical College
Coronary disease, 116
Cortex
relationship to basal ganglia, 54
effects of drugs on, 54
relation to labyrinth, 89
investigations of, 107
Cortical electrical potentials, 135
Cortical relations of the rage reaction, 89
Craig test of syphilis, 135
Cranial pressure, relation to clinical diagnostic procedure, 96
Cryptorchidism, 42
Cultural factors, 139
evaluation of, 35
relative to management of sickness, 35
Curare, 39, 122, 130
Cyclic changes, 35

D

Deaf mutes, 97
Deafness, 94
Death, children's reactions to, 129
Delinquencies, diagnosis and classification of, 41
Delinquency, juvenile, prevention, 116

Delinquent youth, new legal process for, 58
Delinquents
juvenile, study of, 45
juvenile, diagnostic and treatment service, 58
juvenile, mental deviations in, 97
solitary, study of, 58
Delirium, 52
Delirium tremens,
insulin treatment, 110
sodium chloride in treatment of, 124
Delvinol, 86
Dementia praecox, see Schizophrenia
Depressions
electrical potential in the hypothalamus in, 66
classification of, 129
Dermatitis, 49
Dermatitis, Atrophic, emotional influences in, 94
Detroit, Mich., research projects, 28–30, 108–9
Detroit (Mich.), Harper Hospital, see Harper Hospital
Detroit (Mich.), Henry Ford Hospital, see Henry Ford Hospital
Development, normal and atypical, films on, 81
Development and growth, relation to inter-personal and situational experiences, 117
Diagnostic procedure, cranial pressure in relation to, 96
Diagnostic techniques, 127
Diagnostic tests, 41
Dilantin, 73, 86
Disabilities, Educational, 41
Disease
mental and personality disturbances accompanying, 46
processes, effects of, 54
structural, effects on growth, 55
physical, psychological concomitants, 56
social and emotional components in, 96
Diseases, Infectious, induced fever in treatment of, 39

Heredity—Continued
  relation to prognosis in dementia praecox, 65
  in behavior deviations, 76
  relation to dementia praecox, 106, 107
  in drug addiction, 135
Hillman Hospital, Birmingham, Ala., 72
Hillside Hospital, New York
  report of research projects, 112
  list of current research projects, 159
  research personnel, 181
  financial support, 197
Hobbies of young neurotics, 58
Holy Cross Hospital, Chicago, 67
Homer G. Phillips Hospital for Negroes, St. Louis, Mo., 90
Homicide, 29
Homosexuals, 111–12
Hormonal changes in women, 69
Hormone therapy, 133
Hormones, anti-insulin, isolation and application in dementia praecox, 67
Hospital
  administrative problems, 128
  as a community institution, 140
  its value to research, 140
Hospitals, Mental, number of patients in, 1
Hospitals, Private
  proprietary and voluntary, compared, 21–22
Huntington's Chorea, 64
Hydrogen ion concentration, 64
Hyperactivity in children, 133
Hyperinsulinism, experimental, 64
Hyperpyrexia, 64
Hypertension, 45, 69, 91, 94, 116, 128
Hyperventilation
  P. H. in, 49
  psychological aspects in childhood, 66
  with reference to anxiety, 97
Hypnosis, 29, 79, 129
Hypochondriasis, 31

Hypoglycemia
  in tension states, 45
  correlations of blood, alcohol and behavior variations in, 124
Hypophis-ectomized cases, 51
Hypothalamic electrical potentials, 135
Hypothalamic functioning in drug addiction, 135
Hypothalamic functions and emotions, 88
Hypothalamus, 124
  electrical potential in, 66
  hypothalamic region of the brain, 71
Hypothermia, 36, 50
Hysterectomy, 49

I

Illegitimacy, 109
Immaturity, 81
Immunology, 87, 96
Impotence, 88
Individual, Total, 46
Inductotherm, 36
Infancy, early, behavior problems, 106
Infant growth and behavior, 106
Infants, special technique of examining behavior in, 117
Infection, hidden, 138
Infections, 55, 71–72
Influenza, 128
Injuries, experimental, 54
Institute of child welfare, Berkeley, see University of California
Institutes, on problems of adult-child relationships, 128
Institutional placement of children, 126
Institutions, number canvassed, 3–4
Institutions, Private
  compared with public institution, 21
  proprietary and voluntary hospital compared, 21–22
Insulin
  biochemical and clinical studies, 39
  tolerance in dementia praecox, 64
  effect on central nervous system of animals, 64–65
  coma, 99

May Institute for Research, Cincinnati, O., 70, 72
Mayo Clinic, Rochester, Minn., 31
Medical history taking, incorporation of psychiatric elements, 36
Medical practice, personal and situational elements in, 91
Medical problems, internal, psychiatric factors, 45
Medical school centers, list of, 6–7
Medical schools
number canvassed, 4–5
number engaged in research, 14
role of, 22
Medical students, psychiatric education of, 79
Medicine
researches in, 33
internal, problems of, 56–57
psychological, 74
Memory, 26, 91
changes, 123
influence of emotions on, 129
Meningitis, Yeast, 124
Menninger Sanitarium and Clinic and Southard School, Topeka, Kan.
report of research projects, 127–29
list of current research projects, 152–53
research personnel, 175
financial support, 193
Menopausal problems, 116
Menstrual cycle, 69
Mental defectives
school for, 87
racial distribution of admissions to state schools, 102
Mental defects in infancy, 80
Mental deficiency
relation to convulsions, 56
research at Vineland Training School, 131–32
motor disorders in etiology of, 132
paucity of research, 139
Mental development, correlation with pneumoencephalographic findings, 97

Mental deviations in juvenile delinquents, 97
Mental disease
social and biological aspects, 102
expectation and outcome of, 102
Mental disorders
incipient, 41
relation to deficiency of Vitamin B, 72
relation to behavior problems of infancy, 106
Mental hospital survey service, 134
Mental hygiene
program, 46
techniques for prophylactic application of, 46
community aspects, 61
unit for experimental study in, 85
service at kindergarten level, 119
consultant service to state health departments, 134
Mental states, etiological involvement of the auditory apparatus in, 130
Mercy Hospital, Chicago, 67
Mescaline, 106
Metabolic investigations, 35, 69, 87, 90, 123, 134
Metabolism, functions of, 81
Methodist Hospital, Omaha, 39
Methylene blue, 73
Metrazol
use in depressive states, 29, 39
neuropathological manifestations of animals, 44–45
effects, 50
used at Orthogenic school, 62
potassium and calcium during convulsions, 64
effect on central nervous system of animals, 64–65
therapy in functional psychoses, 65
mode of action, 72
experimental use in treatment, 75
follow-up study, 79
treatment, physiochemical studies of spinal fluid, 89
shock therapies, efficacy of, 102

Neurology, experimental, 88, 89
Neurology, vegetative, 47
Neuropathological studies, 30, 36, 54, 71, 96
Neuropathology, 95
training in, 37
resources for, 48, 63, 88
pathological museum, 96
Neurophthalmology, 89
Neurophysics, 106
Neurophysiolpgical studies, 35, 52, 96
Neurophysiology
resources for, 63
of the spinal cord, 106
Neuropsychiatric course, 52–53
Neuropsychiatric problems, 91
Neuropsychiatric studies, 30
Neuropsychiatry, in obstetrics and gynecology, 65
Neuropsychological studies, 91
Neuroses
studies of, 42
production of experimental, 44
elimination in animals, 44
early manifestations, 46
P. H. in hyperventilation in, 49
in relation to Raynaud's disease, 49
relation to effects from frustration, 62
vegetative, 69
anxiety, 88
interpersonal relations underlying, 91
therapy of, 91
experimental, in animals, 91
traumatic, 108, 129
Neurosyphilis, 52, 65
Neurosyphilitic patients, treatment for, 26
Neurotics, care and treatment, 116
Neurotics, young, pursuit of hobbies, 58
New England colleges, survey of psychiatric services offered by, 127
New England Home for Little Wanderers, 57
"New Facts on Mental Disorders," by Neil Dayton, 104
New Haven (Conn.) Children's Community Center, 83

New Haven (Conn.) Community Fund, 82
New Haven, Conn., research projects, 80–83
New Haven Hospital, New Haven, 80, 82
New York City. Board of Education, 119
New York City. Committee for the Study of Sex Variants
report of research projects, 111–12
research personnel, 181
New York City. Community Service Society, 35
New York City, Hillside Hospital, see Hillside Hospital
New York City, Mt. Sinai Hospital, see Mt. Sinai Hospital
New York City, Neurological Institute, 37
New York City, Presbyterian Hospital, see Presbyterian Hospital
New York City, research projects, 32–38, 111–19
New York Hospital—Cornell University Medical College, New York
report of research projects, 32–37
list of current research projects, 160–61
research personnel, 182–83
financial support, 197–98
New York Infirmary for Women and Children, New York
report of research projects, 117–18
list of current research projects, 161
research personnel, 183
financial support, 198
New York Post Graduate Hospital and Medical School, New York
report of research projects, 37–38
list of current research projects, 161
research personnel, 183
financial support, 198
New York School of Social Work, 41, 113
New York State Department of Education, 41
New York State Department of Mental Hygiene, Albany

Psychoanalysis—Continued
effects on patients, 125
application to institutional cases, 129
statistical studies of treatment results, 129
application to preventive work, 129
Psychoanalytic principles in mental hygiene consultation, 129
Psychoanalytic techniques, modified, 129
Psychobiology
studies in, 65
course in, 74
Psychological functions, 81
Psychological growth, 86
Psychological internes, 54
Psychological studies, 37, 65, 85, 86, 129, 135
Psychological testing, 36, 129
devices, applied to Selective Service registrants, 131
Psychological tests
in studying levels of consciousness, 49
standardization of norms of, 58
Psychologists
clinical training, 29
courses for, 95
Psychology, 64
human, 34
teaching resources for students, 61
affective, studies in, 65
clinical, 81
experimental, 81
abnormal, teaching of, 121
topological, 129
Psychometric studies, 117–18
Psychometrics
training of students in, 93, 121
group, 135
Psychoneurosis
therapeutic work with, 40
aid to physicians in handling, 40
services for, 41
records of cases, 45
blood pressure reactions, 64
obsessive compulsion, 120
report of four years of research, 126–27

Psychoneurotic patients
long-term study of, 37
analysis of factors in, 45
provision for, 47
understanding and treatment of, 48
sub-shock treatment, 78
study of, 108
Psychopathic personality, 27, 37, 59
Psychopathology, 34, 96, 135
Psychophysiology, 96
Psychoses (See also Mental disease; Mental disorders)
contrasted with lesser psychopathology, 34
of late-life, 35
relation to effects from frustration, 62
effects of oxygen consumption role in, 64
endocrine therapy, 65
prolonged sleep therapy, 65
symptomatic, treatment of, 65
functional, metrazol therapy in, 65
tissue changes correlated with, 71
personality studies of psychotic persons, 72
interpersonal relations underlying, 91
therapy of, 91
associated with deafness, 94
nutritional deficiencies in, 110
functional, estrogenic substances in, 112
incipient, care and treatment, 116
psychoanalytically oriented treatment, 125
Psychoses, Alcoholic, 41
Psychoses, Arteriosclerotic, 37
Psychoses, Manic depressive
psychoanalysis of, 65
hereditary and environmental factors, 102
Psychoses, Traumatic, 42
Psychosomatic medicine, 139, 144
Psychosomatic studies, 35, 37, 43, 48, 56, 66, 69, 81, 85, 88, 89, 91, 116, 122, 128, 130
Psychotherapeutic procedures, 85
Psychotherapy, 66, 69, 129
Puberty, precocious, 117

HISTORICAL ISSUES IN MENTAL HEALTH

An Arno Press Collection

American Psychopathological Association. **Trends Of Mental Disease.** 1945

Belknap, Ivan. **Human Problems Of A State Mental Hospital.** 1956

Berkley, Henry J. **A Treatise On Mental Diseases.** 1900

Bond, Earl D. **Thomas W. Salmon: Psychiatrist.** 1950

Briggs, L. Vernon. **Two Years' Service On The Reorganized State Board Of Insanity In Massachusetts,** August, 1914 to August, 1916. 1930

Briggs, L. Vernon. **A Victory For Progress In Mental Medicine.** 1924

Burrow, Trigant. **A Search For Man's Sanity.** 1958

Cahow, Clark R. **People, Patients and Politics.** (Doctoral Dissertation, Duke University, 1967). 1979

The Committee of the American Neurological Association for the Investigation of Eugenical Sterilization. **Eugenical Sterilization.** 1936

Cotton, Henry A. **The Defective Delinquent And Insane.** 1921

Dayton, Neil A. **New Facts On Mental Disorders.** 1940

Fein, Rashi. **Economics of Mental Illness.** 1958

Goldhamer, Herbert and Andrew W. Marshall. **Psychosis And Civilization.** 1953

Gosney, E.S., and Paul Popenoe. **Sterilization For Human Betterment.** 1929

Greenblat, Milton, et al. **From Custodial To Therapeutic Patient Care In Mental Hospitals.** 1955

Grob, Gerald N., editor. **Immigrants And Insanity.** 1979

Grob, Gerald N., editor. **Mental Hygiene In Twentieth Century America.** 1979

Grob, Gerald N., editor. **The Mentally Ill In Urban America.** 1979

Grob, Gerald N., editor. **The National Association For The Protection of the Insane And The Prevention Of Insanity.** 1979

Grob, Gerald N., editor. **Psychiatric Research In America.** 1979

Grob, Gerald N., editor. **Psychiatry and Medical Education.** 1979

Grob, Gerald N., editor. **Public Policy And Mental Illness.** 1979

Grimes, John Maurice. **Institutional Care Of Mental Patients In The United States.** 1934

Gurin, Gerald, et al. **Americans View Their Mental Health.** 1960

Hinsie, Leland. **The Treatment Of Schizophrenia.** 1930

Jahoda, Marie. **Current Concepts Of Positive Mental Health.** 1958

Joint Commission On Mental Illness And Health. **Action For Mental Health.** 1961

Koren, John. **Summaries Of State Laws Relating To The Insane.** 1917

Landis, Carney, and James D. Page. **Modern Society and Mental Disease.** 1938

Lewis, Nolan D.C. **Research In Dementia Praecox.** 1936

Malzberg, Benjamin. **Social And Biological Aspects Of Mental Disease.** 1940

May, James V. **Mental Diseases.** 1922

Myerson, Abraham. **Speaking Of Man.** 1950

The National Committee for Mental Hygiene. **State Hospitals In The Depression.** 1934

National Research Council, The Committee on Psychiatric Investigations. **The Problem Of Mental Disorder.** 1934

Plunkett, Richard J. and John E. Gordon,. **Epidemiology And Mental Illness.** 1960

Rapoport, Robert N., et al. **Community As Doctor.** 1960

Robison, Dale W. **Wisconsin And The Mentally Ill.** (Doctoral Dissertation, Marquette University, 1967). 1979

Sicherman, Barbara. **The Quest For Mental Health In America, 1880-1917.** (Doctoral Dissertation, Columbia University, 1967). 1979

Smith, Stephen. **Who Is Insane?** 1916

Stearns, Henry Putnam. **Insanity.** 1883

United States Surgeon General's Office. **The Medical Department Of The United States Army In The World War.** 1929

Wertheimer, F.I., and Florence E. Hesketh. **The Significance Of The Physical Constitution In Mental Disease.** 1926

White, William A. **The Mental Hygiene Of Childhood.** 1919

White, William A. **William Alanson White.** 1938

RC
337
.N32
1980

RC
337
.N32

1980